THE OMEGA-3 ANSWER

A new nutritional medicine

It's natural, it's my health

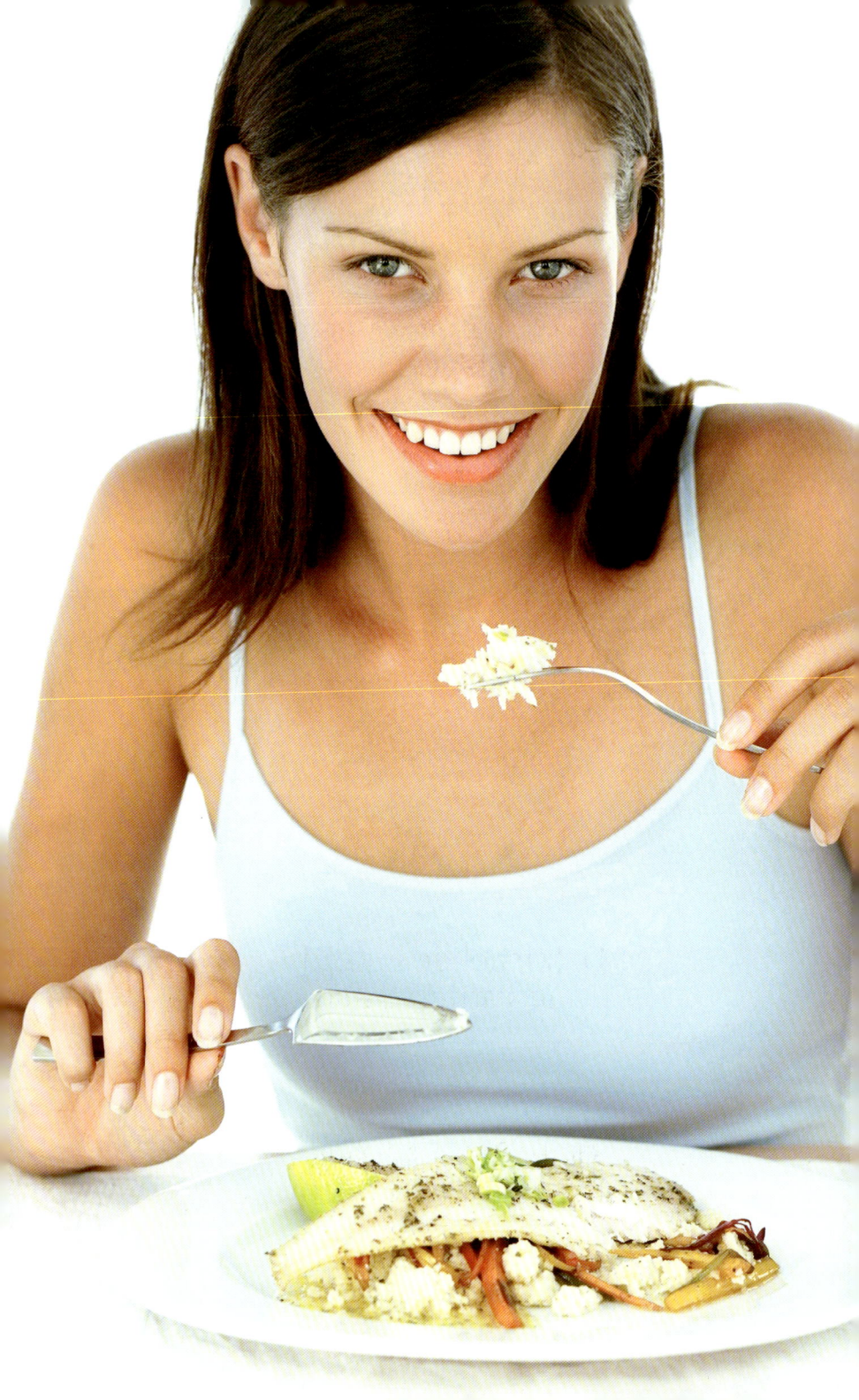

THE OMEGA-3 ANSWER

A new nutritional medicine

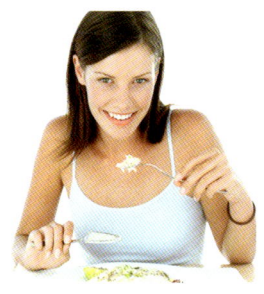

Dr Michel de Lorgeril
and Patricia Salen

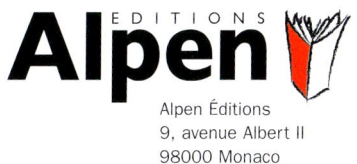

Alpen Éditions
9, avenue Albert II
98000 Monaco

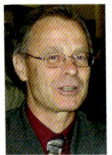
Michel de Lorgeril is a cardiologist, nutritionist and researcher with the (French) National Center for Scientific Research (CNRS). He has worked in the cardiology services of the hospitals of Geneva, Montreal and Lyon. Head of the Experimental Cardiology Laboratories of the Cardiology Institute of Montreal and then of the National Institute for Health and Medical Research (INSERM) in Lyon, he was the main investigator of the well-known Lyon Study and the promoter of scientific concepts such as the *French Paradox* and the Mediterranean diet.

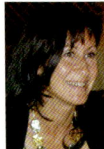
Patricia Salen is a dietician and clinical research assistant.
She is responsible for the nutritional aspects of the Lyon Study and for the dietary programs for heart transplant patients (Lyon, 1989-1996) and heart failure (Saint-Étienne, 1996-1999). She is involved in various research programs in clinical nutrition (primarily European).

Exclusive copyrights:
©Alpen Éditions
9, avenue Albert II
98000 Monaco
Tel: +377 97 77 62 10
Fax: +377 97 77 62 11
web: www.alpen.mc

Printed in Italy
ISBN: 978-2-35934-044-0

Copyrights:
Blue box, Photo Alto, Dynamic graphics, Photo Disc, Stockbyte, Digital Vision, Image 100, Image State, Image Source, Thinkstock, Brand X, Banana Stock, Corbis, Italia Stock, Botanicus, BSIP, Dermatlas, Hemera
Copyright © 20 N. Abdallah and licensers: all rights reserved.

All rights reserved. No part of this publication may be reproduced, stored in a retrieval system, or transmitted in any form or by any means, electronic, electrostatic, magnetic tape, mechanical, photocopying, recording or otherwise, without prior permission in writing from the publisher.

Introduction

The great medical and scientific discovery of the end of the last century was certainly that cardiovascular diseases, scourge of the 20th Century and worse even than the medieval plague, are the result of a recent and ill-conceived evolution in our way of life. Because the 20th Century was also the era of notable technological progress (in transport, agriculture, chemistry, pharmacy, health), which has considerably lengthened our life expectancy, this disengagement of man from his environment has become apparent only in recent times. For example, in the 1960s-1970s (at a time when the principal infectious diseases seemed to be defeated thanks to antibiotics and vaccinations), the cause of death for one in two Americans was cardiac crisis, occurring generally around the age of fifty - at the prime of life!

Our explanation during the 1980s was that the dietary habits of these populations were the main cause of this misfortune. Certainly, other factors were involved (smoking, sedentary lifestyle), but these were probably secondary. Some populations, after all (example the Japanese), present few cardiovascular pathologies despite a very high tobacco consumption. This may be explained by the fact that they generally maintained their traditional eating habits. They gave in to the Marlboro cigarette but they kept well away from Kentucky Fried Chicken!

The reasons, therefore, were related primarily to changes in eating habits. But solid arguments were required to support this theory! The specific aim of the

WARNING:

The information contained in this book is not a substitute for expert advice. Please consult a doctor or a qualified pharmacist before any resort to self-medication.

Lyon Diet Heart Study, conducted in France, was to show that patients having a high risk of cardiac crisis (heart attack) could significantly alter their prognosis if they modified their eating habits (and reverse the process, so to speak, by which their disease arose and progressed). These cardiac patients, picked at random, were required to adopt a so-called "Mediterranean" diet enriched in omega-3 fatty acids. The control group was required to follow a diet normally recommended to cardiac patients. After four years, the risk of repeat cardiac crisis had diminished by 70% in the experimental group; results which exceeded our expectations. Not only were the results of this study confirmed by other research, but since then they have served as a reference point for various national medical academies (notably American and European), for all "heart and nutrition" practitioners and consequently for all their patients as well. This study also created a whole new world for researchers, the "magic world of omega-3s" which we will endeavor to describe in this book.

"Magical" because each day we are discovering new medical applications of the idea of "deficiency in and lack of omega-3", which appears to characterize western populations (from cardiology to psychiatry, through neonatology, oncology and diabetology). What emerges today from looking (as only medicine can do) at the broader spectrum of pathologies activated or encouraged by this simple nutritional deficiency, is the idea that we have both naively and profoundly altered our environment during recent decades and that we are only now beginning to appreciate the serious consequences of this for human health.

TABLE OF CONTENTS

INTRODUCTION ... 5

THE WORLD OF OMEGA-3s ... 10
- **Introducing fatty acids** ... 12
- **Why are we deficient in omega-3?** ... 14
- **How our cells utilize fatty acids** ... 16
- **Derivatives of fatty acids** ... 18

FROM FACTS TO HYPOTHESES: ORIGIN OF THE "DISEASES OF CIVILIZATION" ... 20
- **The geography of health** ... 20
- **Cholesterol does not explain everything** ... 22
- **Excessive pace of nutritional change** ... 24
- **What is the role of genetics?** ... 26
- **From cardiovascular diseases to obesity and diabetes** ... 28

COMBATING CARDIOVASCULAR ILLNESSES WITH OMEGA-3s ... 30

CARDIOVASCULAR DISEASES: WHO IS WORRIED? ... 32
- **The epidemiological data** ... 32
- **The eloquent example of the Eskimos** ... 34
- **Protective yes, but at what dose?** ... 36
- **When the data go against the current** ... 38

CARDIOVASCULAR DISEASES: WHAT HAPPENS WHEN YOU COMPENSATE FOR OMEGA-3 DEFICIENCIES?   40

    Better than drugs   40
    The DART study   42
    The Lyon study in France   44
    Lessons from the Lyon study   46
    The GISSI study   48
    The advent of the Mediterranean diet   50
    New evidence   52

CARDIOVASCULAR DISEASES: HOW DO OMEGA-3s PROTECT THE HEART?   54

    Three protective effects   54
    And alpha-linolenic acid?   56
    Open competition between omega-3 and omega-6   58
    Other potential protective mechanisms   60

PREVENT CANCER WITH OMEGA-3s   62

    Breast cancer   64
    Colon and rectal cancers   66
    From Los Angeles to Lyon: the clinical studies   68
    From Los Angeles to Lyon: the conclusions   70

OMEGA-3S IN INFLAMMATORY DISEASES   72

    When the immune system errs   72
    Painful joints   74
    Rheumatoid arthritis   76
    To prevent asthma   78
    When asthma has taken hold   80
    Protecting oneself against Alzheimer's disease   82

TABLE OF CONTENTS

When the colon is the seat of the inflammation	84
An inflammatory skin disease: psoriasis	86
Osteoporosis, an inflammatory bone disease	88
When insulin resists	90
Obesity: From paradox to catastrophe!	92

OMEGA-3S FOR THE BRAIN… 94

… of the baby	94
… of the mother	96
The revolution of omega-3s in psychiatry	98
An illness of society: depression	100
Counter depression by eating fish	102
The other psychiatric illnesses	104
Omega-3s for better sight	106

OMEGA-3 PROGRAM 108

More omega-3 of vegetable origin	108
Other sources of ALA	110
More omega-3 of marine origin	112
How to enrich one's food intake with omega-3 fatty acids?	114
Less omega-6	116
The Mediterranean diet, a model to follow	118

CONCLUSION 120
GLOSSARY 121
BIBLIOGRAPHY 123

THE WORLD OF OMEGA-3s

Fats (lipids), including those present in foods, are important in medicine because they form the structural basis of our cell membranes and they have an impact on cell functions crucial to our health. The two principal lipid molecules are cholesterol and fatty acids.

Cholesterol excites considerable interest in medicine while, curiously, fatty acids are relatively neglected even though, in mass and complexity, lipids are the most important living organisms.

Cholesterol: what you need to know

Cholesterol is a specifically animal molecule, absent from plants. The description of the way in which the body manufactures cholesterol was the subject of an intense paper chase among biologists during the last century, and several were awarded the Nobel prize for their efforts. Cholesterol is the precursor to numerous hormones (involved in the reproduction and therefore survival of the species) and it is required for the absorption of food fats because it enables the formation of bile.

For all these reasons, and also because it can be easily measured in the blood using simple techniques, cholesterol dosage was - along with that of glucose - the first biological dosage systematically used in

No freedom for our lipids

Lipids are molecules which are adverse to water, in other words they do not dissolve in water. To be functional, they must therefore organize themselves in a particular way. For example, they are almost never "free" in our principal fluids (the main one being blood) but they associate with other molecules or they organize themselves into more or less complex molecular structures, right up to the formation of membranes.

medicine to try and understand and prevent cardiovascular diseases.

Anti-cholesterols: overestimated efficacy

The discovery that high cholesterol is statistically associated with the risk of heart attack has led to intensive research into foods and anti-cholesterol medicines. These studies, however, are not without ulterior commercial motives. Some of these medicines can be effective in the prevention of heart attack. Nevertheless, the industrial and commercial stakes here are extremely high, and one is driven to conclude that the benefits of anti-cholesterol medicines (especially regarding life expectancy) have been hyped out of all proportion. As a result of competition between medicines, the commercial advertising of these medicines is sometimes as exaggerated as advertising for washing powders.

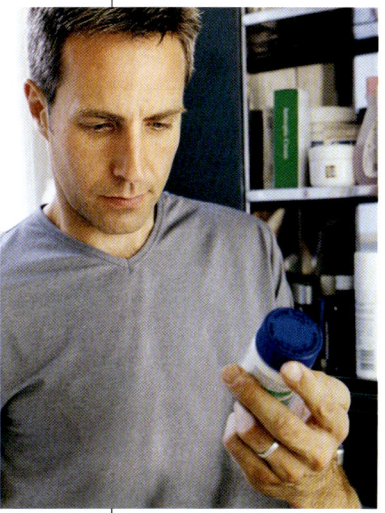

No adequate scientific data exist, however, on the value of anti-cholesterol medicines for populations (Asiatic or Mediterranean) which have never been tested on them, although they represent a considerable expense entry for health insurance. One hopes that this squandering of money will be corrected and that a way of reconciling business, scientific rationality and public health will soon be found!

Introducing fatty acids

Fatty acids are fundamental to the life of simple organisms (bacteria) or complex organisms (mammals) because they structure all biological membranes, forming a "fluid mosaic", each small piece of which is a fatty acid!

Saturated and unsaturated

Fatty acids are simple linear combinations of carbon atoms with an acid function at one extremity. They are connected to molecules, cholesterol and glycerol *(see box)*, which neutralize the acid function.

Fatty acids determine the properties of cells. Some also serve as messengers (like hormones) between tissues or cells and help protect us from attack, especially of the infectious variety. Finally, fatty acids are fuel for our muscles and when one consumes more than necessary they are stored in the adipose tissue.

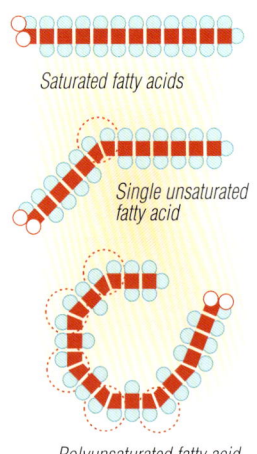

Saturated fatty acids

Single unsaturated fatty acid

Polyunsaturated fatty acid

Fatty acids may be distinguished according to the number of carbon atoms and the type of connection that exists between these atoms (simple or double). Indeed it is this which determines the general form of the molecule and its properties, particularly when it is present in a biological membrane. Therefore, there are fatty acids with short chains (less than 18 carbons), long chains (18 carbons) and very long chains (20 to 24 carbons).

It is customary to classify fatty acids by reference to the existence or otherwise of unsaturated carbon atoms (where one of the atom's electrons fails to couple), giving rise to what is called a double bond between two carbon atoms. To be distinguished:
- **saturated** fatty acids: no double bond
- **unsaturated** fatty acids: one or more double bonds

Unsaturated fatty acids may in turn be classified according to the number of double bonds present. Those with a single double bond are called monounsaturates, such as the oleic acid in olive oil. Those with several double bonds are called polyunsaturates, such as linoleic acid (two double bonds) in canola and sunflower oils.

From omega-3s to omega-9s

Finally, among polyunsaturated fatty acids, the position of the first double bond on the carbon chain allows the family to be identified. If the first double bond occurs at carbon atom no. 3, then we have omega-3 fatty acids (found mostly in flax oil or fatty fish). In addition to omega-3s, there are also omega-6s, omega-7s and omega-9s. Omega-9 - oleic acid - (abundant in olive and canola oil) has only one double bond at carbon atom no. 9. This fatty acid is very resistant (to oxygen, to heat and to ultraviolet), it reflects the physical characteristics of the olive tree and its resistance to the climatic constraints it is subject to. Human cells are capable of synthesizing all saturated fatty acids, as well as oleic acid. Omega-7s are more characteristic of dairy products (result of the process of rumination). Man is not able to synthesize fatty acids with 18 carbon atoms of the omega-3 and omega-6 series: they are said to be "essential".

Fatty acids	Primary food sources
Saturated	Animal products (butter, cream, meat, cold cuts, cheese) Tropical oils (palm, coconut) Cocoa butter, pastries
Monounsaturated	Olive, rapeseed and peanut oils Hazelnut, almond, pistachio Avocado
Polyunsaturated	**Omega-3** Oils from rapeseed, walnut, soy, flax, wheat germ Certain green leaf vegetables Fatty fish (sardines, mackerel, tuna, salmon, etc.)
	Omega-6 Oils from sunflower, corn, soy, hazelnut, sesame, canola, safflower

Reviving medical biology

When the results of a blood sample are returned to the laboratory, they only give the proportion of cholesterol and of glycerol (imprecisely indicated by the term "triglycerides") - no attention is paid to fatty acids. This form of medical biology is somewhat archaic because it neglects the principal lipids of living organisms.

Why are we deficient in omega-3?

Principally because the food produced by modern agriculture and agribusiness has significantly declined in quality over recent decades. But it is a complicated story and requires some introductory remarks.

Essential fatty acids are crucial to the functioning of many living organisms and, for human beings, they are required for optimal health. They may be compared to vitamins: in the same way, our deficiency in them may be absolute or relative, but it can also be quite serious.
Officially, there are only two essential fatty acids *(see box)*:
• linoleic acid, omega-6,
• alpha-linolenic acid (ALA), omega-3.
We are in theory capable of synthesizing their more complex descendents (longer, more double bonds) which are very important for human health, such as eicosapentaenoic and docosahexaenoic acids (EPA and DHA) of the omega-3 family.
In reality, our capacities for synthesis are limited, especially at the extremities of life *(see box)*. **We depend on nutrition for our supply of the whole omega-3 series, and not just for our supply of alpha-linolenic acid, the first in the series.**

> ### Limited capacities for synthesis
>
> Certainly, our cells transform alpha-linolenic acid into EPA. However the transformation of EPA into DHA is disputed by numerous biochemists. In other words, we probably do not know how to manufacture sufficient DHA from precursor fatty acids.

In concrete terms, our food should include (in addition to alpha-linolenic acid) foods which are rich in fatty acids with very long omega-3 chains: EPA and DHA. They are to be found almost exclusively in fatty fish or even in fish-oil capsules, and also in eggs from chickens fed on flaxseed. It may also be found in certain offal, such as brain, but this kind of consumption has plummeted since the "mad cow" fiasco.

Too much linoleic acid

Finally, since the essential fatty acids (linoleic and alpha-linolenic) are supplied through our nutrition alone, they should be consumed in **well-balanced quantities** because in order to transform them into composites with longer chains, our cells have recourse to the same biological pathways and the same enzymes, and excessive amounts of one will inhibit metabolism of the other.

A consensus exists today that our nutrition is far too rich in omega-6 linoleic acid and far too poor in omega-3 alpha-linolenic acid.
In other words, we should reduce our intake of linoleic acid (by firstly reducing our consumption of oils from sunflower, corn, soy, grape seeds) and increase our intake of alpha-linolenic acid (oils from canola , nuts, flaxseed).

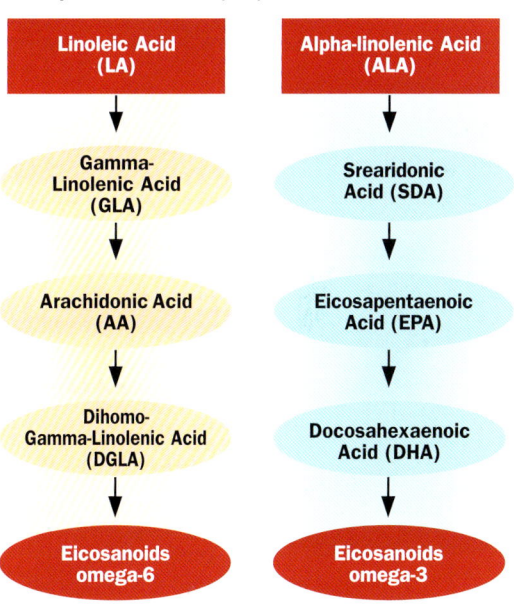

Simplified linoleic acid metabolism (LA) and Alpha-linolenic Acid (ALA)

Essential, what does that mean?

The chemical formula for **linoleic acid** is 18:2 n-6 (or 18:2 omega6) because it has 18 atoms of carbon and 2 double bonds, the first of which occurs at carbon no. 6. That of alpha-linolenic acid (ALA) is 18:3 n-3 (or 18:3 omega-3) because it has 18 carbon atoms and 3 double bonds, the first of which occurs at carbon no. 3. Since our cells are unable to establish double bonds at carbon atoms 3 and 6, linoleic and alpha-linolenic acids cannot be obtained from any other fatty acid. Since they are crucial to human health, they are said to be essential and we must obtain them each day through nutrition.

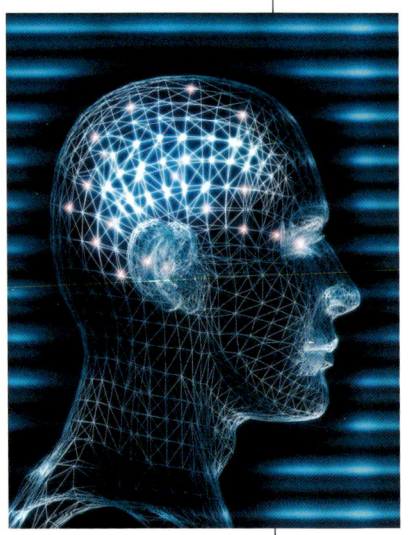

How our cells utilize fatty acids

Absorbed by the intestine, fatty acids can serve as an energy source for muscles, they can be stored in the form of fats or play a direct role in the life of cells by being incorporated in cell membranes.

Fuel and energy reserve

After prolonged fasting, we go into our fatty reserves. Fatty acids, therefore, are both indispensable for our daily activities (muscular activity, internal temperature regulation) and they act as a kind of storeroom for our food surplus.

But the importance of fatty acids for our health is primarily due to the fact that they are the constituents of our cell membranes; these membranes isolate the cell from the surrounding environment and allow the cell to create functional units from within (mitochondria, nucleus).

The concentration of omega-3 fatty acids in our cell membranes (especially of the heart and brain) determines the proper functioning of these organs and their resistance to particular stress situations.

The brain is a mass of lipids

Some organs are particularly rich in fatty acids, independently of their function as a source of energy; for example the brain or the thymus. Over 50 % of brain mass consists of lipids and more than 60 % of these lipids are omega-3 fatty acids.

THE WORLD OF OMEGA-3s

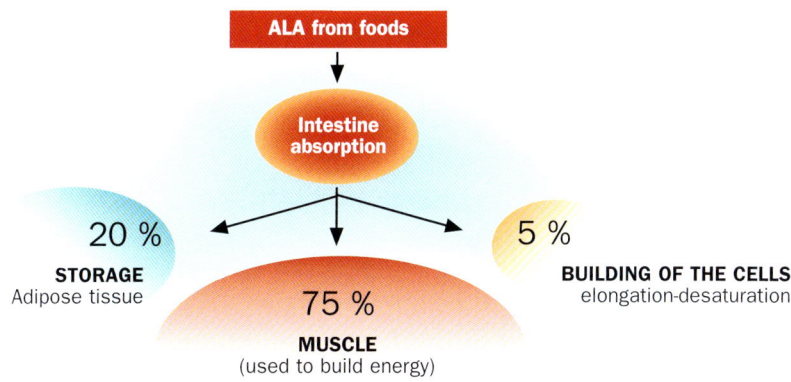

What happens to alpha-linolenic acid (ALA) within the organism
According to estimates produced by studies using radioactive markers, around 75% of the alpha-linolenic acid absorbed is consumed by the muscles to produce energy, 15 to 20% is stored in the adipose tissue (energy reserves) and less than 5% is used by cells.

More efficient cells

The varied activity of many cells depends on the fatty acid composition of their membranes. For example, where there is vascular rupture, blood platelets produce clots which prevent hemorrhages. However they are more or less "reactive" depending on the concentration in their membrane of omega-3 fatty acids.

Another example is the electrical activity of cardiac cells, on which cardiac rhythm depends. This electrical activity is variable, depending on the omega-3s present in the membrane.

Finally, brain cells are very responsive to omega-3s present in their membrane. Certain psychiatric illnesses, or simply one's mood in particular situations (a mother after childbirth, for instance) are strongly associated with omega-3 concentration in the brain.

More resistant neurons

Neurons are better able to withstand lack of oxygen (for instance in a cerebral vascular accident) or other onslaughts (especially due to medicines) when their membranes are enriched by omega-3.

This issue is the subject of fascinating research by the team of Michel Lazdunski in Nice, France, with potential repercussions for medical and surgical neurology.

Derivatives of fatty acids

Fatty acids become integrated in the cell membrane, then some are transformed as required into more complex derivatives: longer-chain fatty acids or messenger molecules such as thromboxanes, prostaglandins or leucotrienes.

More or less powerful messengers

"Essential" fatty acids or their descendents give rise to signaling molecules which serve as messengers. The biological activity of these messengers varies depending on the fatty acids from which they derive. Thus, the messengers that derive from arachidonic acid (omega-6 family) are very active. They encourage the formation of clots and are therefore highly dangerous for coronary patients, who must take aspirin every day to neutralize the arachidonic acid, with consequent risk of hemorrhagic complications, especially of a digestive nature.

On the other hand, messengers derived from EPA (omega-3 fatty acid competitor of arachidonic acid) are less active in the formation of clots and therefore are of little danger to the cardiac patient. Furthermore, EPA prevents heart rhythm disorders and contains anti-inflammatory properties.

Therefore our blood and tissues must contain sufficient concentrations of omega-3 fatty acids to ensure protection against cardiovascular diseases or the arrhythmic complications associated with them.

A double-edged sword

When a hemorrhage occurs, the recruitment of platelets to stop the bleeding is performed by messengers which stimulate the adhesion and aggregation of platelets. Unfortunately, these same messengers may be partly responsible for the formation of clots during a heart attack at the site of an ulcerated atheroma.

Omega-6 and omega-3: competition

Essential omega-6 and omega-3 fatty acids utilize the same biochemical pathways to generate the most complex fatty acids of their respective series. Competition therefore exists between the two series of fatty acids to produce the synthesis of their descendants. Because the latter have different characteristics and different effects on the various processes implicated in the major pathologies (cardiovascular, cancerous, inflammatory and psychiatric), this competition is of fundamental importance in medicine.

In practice, and in the light of current dietary habits, that means that we should reduce our intake of omega-6 fatty acids (linoleic acid and arachidonic acid and our consumption of foods rich in them) and increase our intake of omega-3 fatty acids, if necessary resorting to capsules.

Rather than setting an absolute value for a particular person's intake of omega-3 and omega-6 fatty acids (x grams per day), more important are the relevant ratios (the balance); in other words what matters are the relative quantities of one to the other.

The ratio of omega-6/omega-3 fatty acids should be lower than 4 to 1; according to some scientists it should be as low as 2 to 1.

To find out more:
Cyclooxygenase

The "messenger" molecules which are the descendants of fatty acids are synthesized by the action of several enzymatic systems, including that of cyclooxygenase (or COX). This enzyme owes its renown to the fact that it is completely blocked by aspirin. Aspirin and the other non-steroid anti-inflammatories ease pain and lessen inflammation in large part because they block the COX enzyme and therefore the production of derivatives of arachidonic acid, the principal omega-6 of cell membranes. The partial replacement of arachidonic acid by an omega-3 (EPA) attenuates the inflammatory response without eliminating it. Another medical application of derivatives generated by the COX enzyme is the use by obstetricians of prostaglandins to open the neck of the uterus during a difficult childbirth. This gives an idea of the physiological importance and potential clinical impact of fatty acids transformed by this enzyme.

Indeed, it's a bit more complicated than this because there are two COXs: COX-1, permanently active, and COX-2, said to be "inducible" because it becomes active only during inflammation. One might have thought that medicines which only block COX-2 could be equally effective as COX blockers but without harmful effects for the stomach. Unfortunately, it turns out that the anti-COX-2 increase the risk of cardiovascular diseases (by a mechanism currently poorly understood) and some of these medicines have already been withdrawn from the market.

FROM FACTS TO HYPOTHESES:
ORIGIN OF THE "DISEASES OF CIVILIZATION"

Eating and drinking

Analysis of the dietary habits of populations is extremely complex and has given rise to extraordinary epidemiological studies, notably in relation to cardiovascular illnesses. Several nutritional factors have been cited to explain their protective effect, including consumption of fruit and vegetables, wine or non-refined cereals.

Others factors have been pointed to for their harmful effect, including consumption of dairy products (especially butter and cream), fatty meats and cold cuts as well as excessive amounts of sodium (salt).

The geography of health

Analysis of the frequency of certain illnesses in different countries reveals significant variation from one geographic zone to the other. This is the concept of biogeography.

Certain zones have been and remain overwhelmed by very high cardiovascular mortality: the United-States, Canada and Northern Europe, although there are noticeable exceptions such as Iceland where the rate of cardiovascular mortality is one of the lowest in Europe. Other areas have been spared for a long time, such as Mediterranean Europe or Asia (notably Japan). Similar tendencies apply in respect to forms of cancer, psychopathies, asthma and some inflammatory or metabolic diseases, with resulting wide disparities in life expectancy.

It is unlikely that climatic or socio-economic features explain these disparities. Indeed, some Nordic regions (Iceland, Greenland) are spared, whereas sub-tropical zones (such as Florida or Southern California) or regions in southern Europe (Romania, Bulgaria, Malta) are severely affected by cardiovascular diseases and cancer. Similarly, highly developed countries are either badly affected (United States, Scandinavia) or relatively unaffected (Japan, France, Iceland), while relatively poor countries or those in financial crisis are either badly affected (Russia, Azerbaijan) or protected (China, India). Having said that, geographic differences

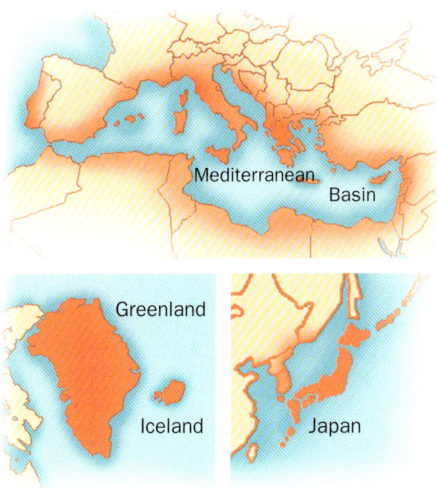

Zones protected from cardiovascular diseases

Omega-3s in the limelight

Careful analysis of the eating habits of protected populations (Japan, Mediterranean region, Iceland, Greenland) shows that they share something in common: high consumption of omega-3 fatty acids of marine or vegetable origin.

appear to be disappearing, as lifestyles around the planet are becoming homogenized - an effect of so-called globalization.

The "French paradox"

Differences in risk levels associated with different geographic zones cannot, therefore, be explained without going beyond an analysis of climatic or socio-economic conditions.

The same question was raised in relation to countries such as France or Switzerland, where the prevalence of cardiovascular diseases is relatively low when compared with neighboring countries. In actual fact, these neighboring countries have comparable climates, socio-economic status and risk profiles (average cholesterol, average blood pressure, prevalence of diabetes, smoking).

This phenomenon may be termed the **French paradox**, and the most credible explanation (or at least partial explanation) for this relates to the consumption of wine.

In relation to the **general idea** of biogeography, the only theory which to date has not been refuted declares that the dietary habits (including drinking habits) of populations is of key explanatory importance. Many scientists hold that only differences in the eating and drinking habits of populations can account for these geographic **variations**.

Cholesterol does not explain everything

Using the geography of health to explain the appalling epidemic of cardiovascular diseases which marked the 20th Century tends to relativize the role of supposedly "traditional" risk factors such as cholesterol and high blood pressure.

The graphs opposite show that the role played by cholesterol and blood pressure in cardiovascular diseases is a relative one. These data are drawn from the largest international epidemiological study every carried out on dietary habits and cardiovascular diseases: the Seven Countries study.

This study provides information of a comparative nature on the relation between increased cholesterol or blood pressure and the risk of death from heart attack. A northern European or an American with a given level of cholesterol or blood pressure has a much higher risk of dying from heart attack than someone from Japan or the Mediterranean region. For northern Europeans and Americans, the risk increases noticeably with the rise in cholesterol and blood pressure levels, while for the others, the risk does not increase at all (Japanese) or increases only slightly (Mediterranean populations). And yet, risk factors including (but not limited to) age, weight and tobacco consumption were similar in the populations studied.

> ### To prescribe is easier
>
> The impact of cholesterol and high blood pressure can be properly understood only in a context which gives due weight to nutritional factors. It is certainly easier (though no less costly in the end) to measure cholesterol and blood pressure than to evaluate one's dietary habits; and it is easier to prescribe tablets afterwards than to try and change the dietary habits of a patient or indeed of his or her family.

Everything depends on dietary habits

At the time of research, the only factor which enabled one to differentiate the various geographic groups and their risk of dying from heart attack was their dietary habits. This means that nutritional factors strongly predominate in the risk of heart attack in different populations.

FROM FACTS TO HYPOTHESES: ORIGIN OF THE "DISEASES OF CIVILIZATION"

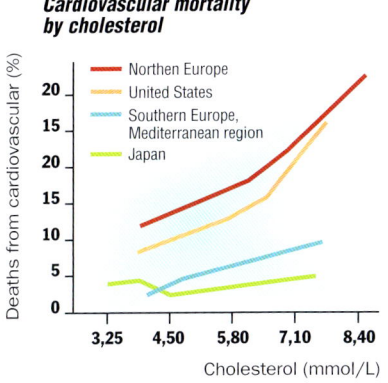

Cardiovascular mortality by cholesterol

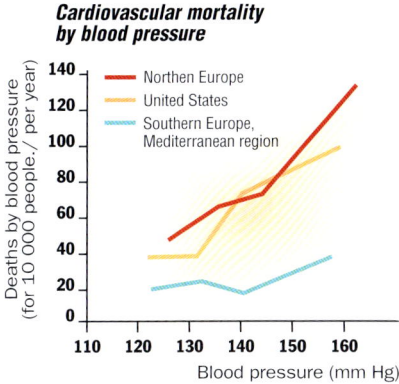

Cardiovascular mortality by blood pressure

Any prevention strategy for heart attack and its complications should as a matter of absolute priority begin by altering the dietary habits of those at risk.

These geographic variations in risk are, moreover, recognized by European medical and scientific authorities which, in their official Recommendations for the *prevention of cardiovascular diseases*, emphasize that the risks (from parameters such as cholesterol and blood pressure) should be calculated according to different criteria for high-risk populations (United States, Northern Europe) or low risk populations (Japan, Mediterranean region). Unfortunately these recommendations are not much observed in practice. Doctors, subject to shrewd and biased marketing from the pharmaceutical industry, handle anti-cholesterol (or anti-high blood pressure) medicines in the same way, irrespective of the country concerned.

Use or Abuse of Cholesterol Drugs in the U.S.

In many industrialized countries around the world, anti-cholesterol and other medicines are over prescribed if not, indeed, abused. In 2001, the U.S. National Institutes of Health, through its national cholesterol education program, issued new clinical practice and management guidelines designed to lower cholesterol levels. If these guidelines were correctly followed, an estimated 36 million Americans (about 18% of American adults) were expected to receive cholesterol lowering drugs, up from 13 million in 2001. France is another country where this is happening. It is estimated that 2 to 3 out of 10 French adults regularly take these medicines.

Excessive pace of nutritional change

Some researchers refer today to a "Paleolithic" diet in their struggle against certain diseases, notably diabetes, obesity and heart attack. What is this all about?

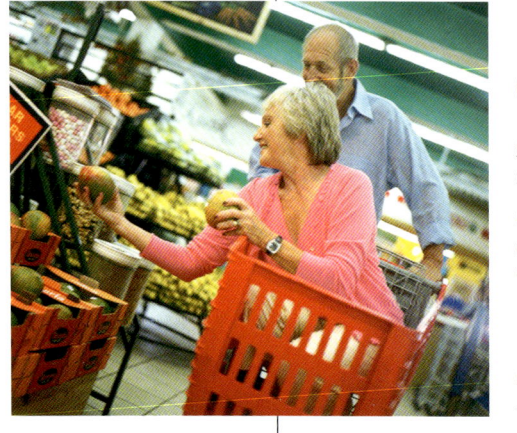

Hunter-gatherers in the supermarket

We are genetically identical to our Paleolithic ancestors (of forty thousand years ago) because according to the rhythm of the genetic clock, forty thousand years is not long enough for significant evolution in our genome. On the other hand, since Paleolithic times our way of life has totally changed. In other words, we are the genetic result of an evolutionary selection which occurred in ancient times (on the scale of millions of years) when our existence was more than precarious (at best we were hunter-gatherers). Today we live with a superabundance of food products and our way of life has become sedentary.

This discordance between our genetically determined ability to withstand the worst conditions of existence and our present highly comfortable way of life (for the majority of us, that is, and by comparison with the lives of hunter-gatherers) in part explains the prevalence of contemporary cardiovascular diseases and metabolic syndromes such as obesity and diabetes.

How did cooking develop?

Some scientists hold that the invention and development of culinary techniques (preparation and heating of food) was actually a strategy invented by Neolithic man to adapt to the harmful consequences to their physiology and health by the consumption of the products of animal breeding and of agriculture, especially cereals and dairy products.

FROM FACTS TO HYPOTHESES:
ORIGIN OF THE "DISEASES OF CIVILIZATION"

Human consumption progress	Pre-human	Hunter-gatherer		Modern man
	- 4 000 000 years	- 100 000 years	1950	2000
Polyunsaturated/saturated rundown	1/1	0.9/1	0.75/1	0.5/1
Omega-6/Omega-3 rundown		1/1	10/1	20/1
Cholesterol		Non-pathogenic	Pathogenic	
Consumption		plants and wild game	Industrial cereals and reared animals	

Without exaggerating this theory, it is arguable that by attempting to emulate the presumed dietary habits of hunter-gatherers (if not their way of life), it might be possible to reduce this discrepancy between our **new** way of life and our **old genes,** thereby reducing the risk of heart attack and the probability that we will become obese or diabetic.

New fats, old genes

The theory that our contemporary nutrition is poorly adapted to our physiology (and to our genetic abilities) has been popularized in the United States by the slogan *new fats, old genes,* the underlying idea being that these new fats are ill-fitted to our old genes.

In actual fact, our organism meticulously organizes our metabolism in accordance with our characteristic genetic abilities and our intake of nutrients. In other words, if we want optimal health then our nutrition must be in harmony with our old genes, which are adapted to the nutrition of hunter-gatherers. This is notably the case with the ratio of omega-6/omega-3 fatty acids, which was quite different in Paleolithic times. One can certainly hope that each of us possesses regulatory systems which help us to compensate, if only partially, for this lack of harmony between our old genes and our new dietary habits. Still, it is better to try and live in harmony with ourselves rather than counting on a hypothetical process of adaptation to protect us from diseases.

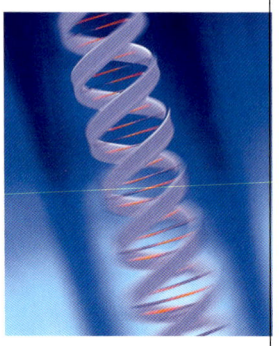

What is the role of genetics?

During the last decade considerable progress has been made in our knowledge of the human genome, creating great hopes for the diagnosis and treatment of chronic illnesses. Up to now, these hopes have been largely disappointing.

Take a Belgian, an Italian and an Englishman...

The general aim of the European study (financed by the European Community) IMMIDIET is to evaluate the impact of dietary habits and genetic variations on the risk profile of four European communities (Flemish in Belgium, Italian in Abruzzo, English in south London and Italo-Belgian in Flanders) at risk of heart attack. The first results clearly indicate that the way of life of these populations (notably their nutrition regime) is of much greater relevance for the determination of risk than genetic characteristics. Paradoxically - but in keeping with the process of homogenization of European populations - it appears that the dietary habits of the English have considerably improved during recent decades, while those of the Italians have deteriorated as a result of losing or forgetting their Mediterranean traditions. These tendencies are accompanied by parallel changes in the prevalence of cardiovascular diseases in these countries, which confirms that protection from risk is not guaranteed by climate or geographical position.

Every doctor knows that there are family predispositions to cardiovascular diseases. The first stage of a medical consultation should consist of questioning the patient about his family's medical history. Still, it is very difficult to know which factor should be given more weight: life habits (changeable) transmitted by the family from generation to generation (and common to a given generation) or a genetic risk (not changeable until proven to the contrary). In fact, the more one studies the links between cardiovascular diseases and the genetic characteristics of individuals, the less weight one gives to genetic factors in comparison with way of life. The so-called "environmental" factors, especially dietary habits, appear to predominate. Should one be surprised? Not really!

FROM FACTS TO HYPOTHESES:
ORIGIN OF THE "DISEASES OF CIVILIZATION"

The health of migrants

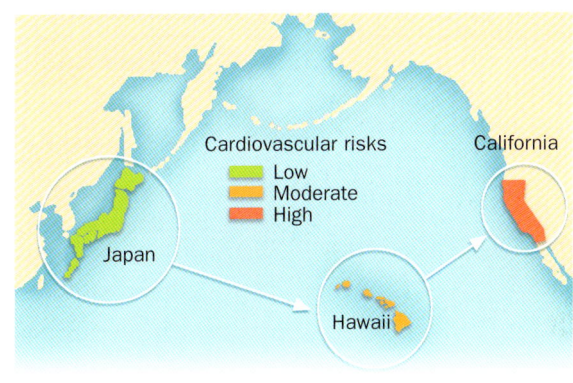

Japanese migration

Studies on migrants, carried out during the years 1960-1970, had already actually suggested that large geographical variations in the incidence of cardiovascular diseases could have neither a genetic explanation nor - all the more so - a racial explanation. Some of these studies remain well-known, especially those relating to Japanese migrants to the United States. This migration generally took place in two stages (in two generations) over the Pacific Ocean. The first generation landed at Hawaii and the second made the big jump from Hawaii to California. Obviously the three populations – the one which remained in Japan, the one from Hawaii and the one from California, are genetically identical. However, cardiovascular risk signaled a noticeable increase among the "new Californians"; it equals the level of risk for indigenous Californians, with whom these immigrants from now on share the same way of life. This risk is at an intermediate level for the "new Hawaiians", according to how they adapt to the American way of life.

However, some migrant populations who preserve their original more protective way of life, shunning their host country's way of life, do not signal an increased risk. This is the case, for instance, with Greek communities in Australia. The determination of many Greek migrants to preserve their traditional way of life has had the effect that some "exiled" communities have remained attached to practices which are no longer in evidence even in contemporary Greece.

From cardio-vascular diseases to obesity and diabetes

No genetic modification can explain the epidemic in heart attack of the 20th Century. The only possible explanation: a change in environmental factors, in first place changes in dietary habits.

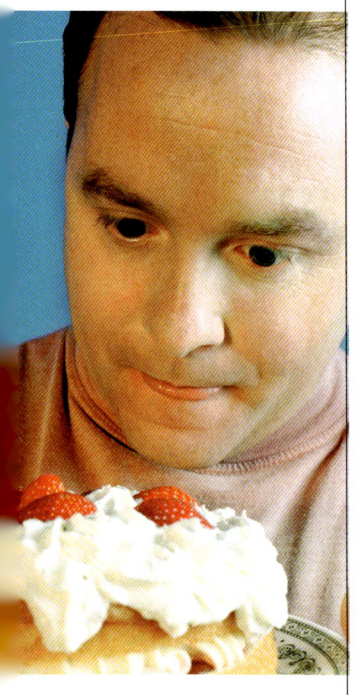

A radical change in dietary habits occurred in the United States just before the war of 1939-1945, and in Europe during the 1950s. The accelerated industrialization of agriculture and breeding, with a parallel decrease in the price of foods of animal origin and the introduction of the cold chain into each home (the refrigerator), resulted in significantly increased consumption of foods of animal origin. It took only one or two decades for butter to cease being a food exclusive to the rich. In the same time, traditional foods were abandoned, either because they were no longer available at an acceptable price (fresh local fruit and vegetables in season, saltwater and freshwater fish), or because they had fallen progressively into disuse (cereals other than wheat, beans and peas of all sorts), at a time when new products flowed in (shortening for French fries, supposedly "light" oils for salads), supported by overbearing publicity campaigns.

FROM FACTS TO HYPOTHESES:
ORIGIN OF THE "DISEASES OF CIVILIZATION"

Outcry against saturated fats

Between 1970 and 1990, there was a significant decline in the **frequency of heart attack**, especially in the United States and Scandinavia. This decline went hand in hand with the decline in consumption of saturated fats of animal origin, especially dairy products. Other factors have certainly had a part to play, but the clinical studies have supported the hypothesis that saturated fats had played a major role in the epidemic, at least between 1930 and 1970. At the same time, an epidemic of metabolic syndromes in these same countries (combination of diabetes, obesity and high blood pressure involving especially the younger generation) has been spreading at an alarming rate since 1990.

How to explain this epidemic conjunction?

In fact, the marked and persistent decline in consumption of **saturated fats** has been offset by a huge increase in **refined carbohydrates** and industrial **polyunsaturated fats** (sunflower, corn, soy) rich in omega-6 fatty acids. These factors taken together promote the development of obesity and diabetes and offer an explanation for the growing prevalence of metabolic syndromes.

Is Europe temporarily protected?

In Europe, where the metabolic syndrome epidemic is not yet as conspicuous as in the United States (one American out of five is thought to have presented with a metabolic syndrome in 2002), the resistance of populations to the "macdonaldization" of dietary habits - in other words a rediscovery of the advantages of traditional dietary habits - could prevent the further spread of the metabolic syndrome epidemic. It could therefore prevent (or at least delay) the new cardiovascular disease epidemic, the worsening of which may be expected as a result of the uncontrolled spread of metabolic syndromes.

The theory of cholesterol

A credible hypothesis is that the decline in consumption of saturated fats occurred through reliance on partially erroneous medical and scientific premises, which may be summarized in one word: the theory of cholesterol. Because no dietary intervention study has ever actually proven that an anti-cholesterol diet, based on high consumption of polyunsaturated vegetable fats, can reduce mortality from heart attack; and the fact that some of these anti-cholesterol diets had promoted the onset of cancers was actually concealed.

COMBATING CARDIO-VASCULAR ILLNESSES WITH OMEGA-3s

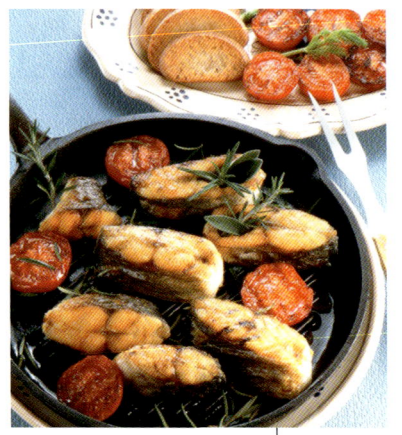

If there is one area of medicine where we can be assured that omega-3s will play a big role, then it's the area of cardiovascular diseases.

Prevention or cure?

These diseases have overwhelmed our society for fifty years; one in three adult men and women or nearly 80 million U.S. adults have some form of cardiovascular disease (estimate extrapolated to U.S. population in 2004 from NHANES 1999-2004). Cardiovascular disease was the underlying cause of death in one of every 2.8 deaths or 36.3% of all deaths in 2004.

Unfortunately, health policies have always favored a remedial approach to these diseases rather than a preventive approach. This generates costs which are obviously significant; equally, of course, it generates profits no less significant for the pharmaceutical industry.

As we saw, these diseases are real nutritional diseases, previously completely unknown to us. Any attempt at dietary prevention must be **comprehensive** and should not be restricted to a single factor, whether a particular medicine or a particular nutrient. It can no longer be doubted that certain types of diets are protective in nature, such as a vegetarian or

Mediterranean diet. These diets are characterized, by and large, by low consumption of fats and animal proteins and high consumption of cereals, fresh and dried vegetables and fresh fruit. However, some nutrients have a special protective effect, among which are **omega-3 fatty acids** of vegetable or marine origin.

The theory of omega-3s, a credible theory

The problems relating to omega-3s perfectly illustrate the way in which a credible (i.e. resistant to criticism) scientific theory arises in medicine *(see box)*. In fact, epidemiologists have clearly shown that we are seriously lacking in omega-3 fatty acids. They have also shown that the risks of developing many diseases (notably cardiovascular) increase with the seriousness of omega-3 deficiency. Clinicians have shown that correcting these deficiencies decreases the risk of occurrence of these diseases, which proves that there is a causal relation between the deficiency and the pathologies. Finally, biologists and physiologists have described several mechanisms which explain how omega-3s are able to withstand these diseases.

Genesis of a scientific theory

For researchers (and doctors) in the area of nutrition and health, a credible scientific theory should rest on three kinds of arguments:

1) **epidemiological observations** (of populations) allowing associations (statistical correspondences) between diseases and nutritional parameters to be studied;

2) **results of randomized clinical trials** (equivalent to drawing lots), comparing an experimental diet with a control diet;

3) studies in **experimental biology** (or physiology), using experimental models (or trials) to examine the biological mechanisms that might explain the epidemiological observations and the results of the clinical trials.

It is the concordance between these three components (epidemiological, clinical and biological) which generates conviction among researchers and thus the credibility (in their eyes) of a scientific theory. However, it is the results of the clinical trials which are most likely to galvanize the medical profession into the prevention (and possibly treatment) of the diseases concerned, even if the scientific facts are not understood in their entirety.

CARDIOVASCULAR DISEASES: WHO IS WORRIED?

The epidemiological data

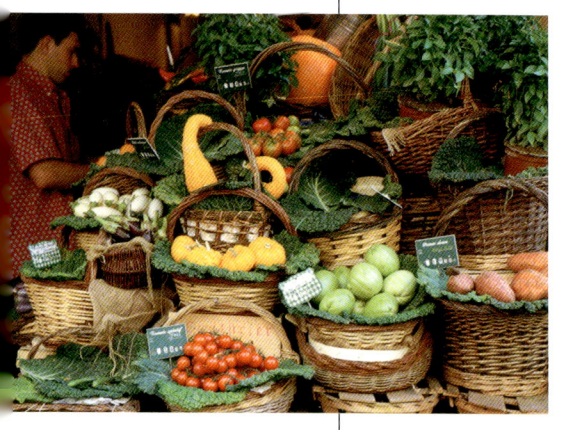

Do correspondences exist between the quantities of omega-3 supplied by nutrition and the cardiovascular state of health of populations? Nutritionists have looked into this question by examining different populations, and their response is a definite yes.

How are the epidemiological data obtained?

With minimal effort and without the need to use patients as subjects of experiment (and the risks this involves), nutritionists are able to obtain important information simply by observing people and their environment. Dietary sources of omega-3 fatty acids vary from one region and population to another, but all human beings have these fatty acids in their blood and in their cells. Of course, the blood and tissue concentrations may vary, in proportion to the quantities present in the foods consumed.

If the dietary habits of a population (or a cohort of patients) is known, as well as the chemical composition (here, the quantities of omega-3) of the main foods consumed, then one can examine whether correspondences exist between the quantity of omega-3 fatty acids ingested and the clinical parameters which show the state of health of this population.

These correspondences are not the result of therapeutic intervention or some other maneuver; they exist in real life, in the natural condition of the human being.

- If the correspondences are strong, they produce crucial information which, where confirmed by clinical trials, can pass directly to clinical practice.
- On the other hand, when these correspondences are weaker, one must resort to complex statistical techniques to make these analyses "speak". In this case, the information must be interpreted with extreme care because other factors may be present which can put the researcher on the wrong track.

Currently available epidemiological data on omega-3 fatty acids and health, especially cardiovascular diseases, are classified as highly significant and do not lend themselves to error.

The more omega-3, the fewer sick people

Whether the researchers used relatively crude nutritional parameters (for instance consumption of fish or marine foodstuffs) or more sophisticated parameters (consumption of actual omega-3 fatty acids) or biomarkers (blood or tissue concentration of one or more omega-3 fatty acids), the analyses conducted at different times and in different regions have, in the great majority of cases, shown that the higher the levels of omega-3, the less frequent and severe are cardiovascular diseases.

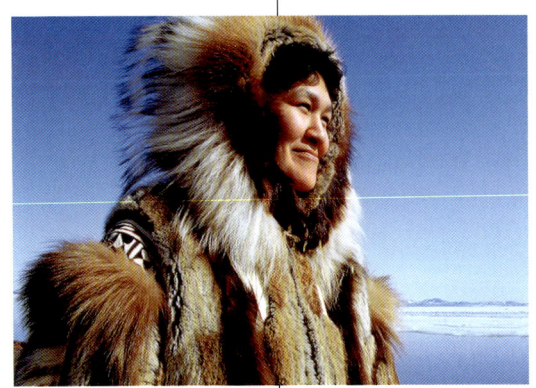

The eloquent example of the Eskimos

It was by observing the way of life and dietary habits of Greenland Eskimos that Danish researchers advanced the hypothesis that omega-3 fatty acids protect the heart.

Why are there omega-3s in cold water fish?

Fish from cold seas require very polyunsaturated fatty acids (like omega-3 fatty acids, EPA and DHA) in their membranes in order to survive in very cold waters poor in oxygen.

The more their membranes contain highly unsaturated fatty acids, the more adaptable (or fluid) they are to a given temperature. At very low temperatures, very long-chain omega-3s can guarantee this membrane fluidity.

This theory has been consolidated by analyses conducted in Japan and in Iceland. The Eskimos, Icelanders and Japanese, in addition to sharing in common a low cardiovascular mortality rate, also have very high concentrations of omega-3 fatty acids in their cell membranes due to the fact that they consume a lot of **fatty fish.**

Some Eskimo communities also obtain their omega-3s from **seal oil** (the seal being a lover of fatty fish, typically found in cold seas).

Seal oil has one advantage over fatty fish. It is relatively rich in monounsaturated fatty acids particularly **resistant to oxygen toxicity** (notably oleic acid, also contained in olive oil). This combination of omega-3 fatty acids and oleic acid is of benefit because it is likely that oleic acid helps to prevent, at least temporarily, the oxidation of omega-3 fatty acids.

Omega-3s in fatty fish, however, are poorly protected against oxygen toxicity because fish inhabit milieus which are by definition poor in oxygen (oceans) and therefore do not require powerful antioxidants to protect themselves.

The Finnish exception

According to epidemiological studies, Finns do not appear to be protected from cardiovascular diseases despite their considerable consumption of fish. A recent explanation by researchers from Helsinki is that fish from Finnish lakes are massively contaminated by heavy metals (especially mercury), which encourage the toxicity of oxygen. In other words, rather than protecting them, Finnish fish poison them.

Since this discovery, it has been shown that several marine species (especially oceanic fish of significant size, among the last links of the oceanic food chain) are contaminated by heavy metals, pesticides, dioxins, so much so that several health authorities are recommending that their affected populations (starting with pregnant women) avoid consuming fish of the high seas such as swordfish and tuna.

A tragic aspect of this story of ocean pollution: it is at the very moment when we are rediscovering the benefits of marine foods for our health that we are coming to understand the extent of the damage caused to marine nature by our industrial and commercial improvidence!

Oxygen toxicity

It is one of the paradoxes of life on Earth: we cannot survive without oxygen but at the same time, this gas is a poison which produces all kinds of pathologies and causes us to grow old! The toxic effects of oxygen make themselves felt through the production of so-called radical substances (free radicals) which are extremely reactive and which modify the structure and function of target molecules. Among the victims of oxygen toxicity are omega-6 and omega-3 fatty acids. This toxicity is in principle checked by "antioxidant defenses".

Protective yes, but at what dose?

Research on homogenous populations such as American nurses or doctors has shown that those who consume the most omega-3 are less affected by cardiovascular diseases. And it has shown the approximate intake required in order to be protected.

The results taken as a whole are remarkable. Small differences in the daily intake of omega-3 lead to considerable differences of risk in the long term. This affects men as well as women, and affects all ages. Moreover, it is in the cardiac and vascular risks where notable reductions have been observed: heart attack, sudden death syndrome or cerebral vascular accident. All patients appear to be protected by omega-3s, whether or not they have already had a cardiac crisis. One very important point, still poorly understood even among researchers, is that all omega-3 fatty acids give protective effect - those of vegetable origin (alpha-linolenic acid or ALA) as well as very long-chain omega-3s of marine origin (EPA and DHA). Some of these studies have enabled us to know what intake of omega-3-rich foods is required to obtain this cardiovascular protection.

Intake of very long-chain omega-3 fatty acids (EPA and DHA) corresponding to the consumption of two to three servings of fatty fish per week appears to give minimal but significant protection.

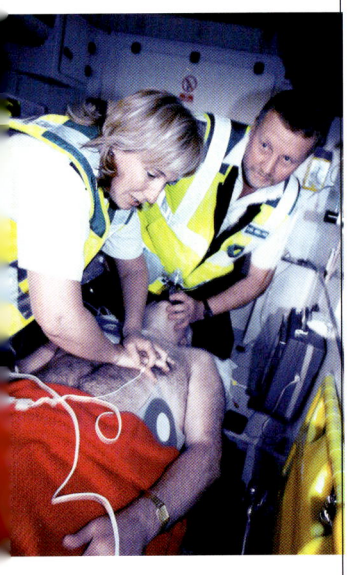

More and more, a dose-effect relation (suggesting that the more one eats, the more one is protected) has shown up in the majority of studies, for a dose of less than two grams per day approximately, which is a strong argument for a causal connection.

The experts appear to agree that the minimum required dose for cardiovascular prevention should be at least 1 g of EPA+DHA per day.

But higher doses are necessary for some patients, especially diabetics, or in order to reduce the risk to even lower and safer levels. Actually, Japanese adults (who have the lowest rate of cardiovascular diseases in the world) consume fish an average of twice a day.

What about alpha-linolenic acid?

For this fatty acid, the epidemiological data are less clear. It is actually the precursor of EPA in the chain of synthesis of omega-3s; therefore it is difficult to account for the protective effects due specifically to ALA and to other omega-3s (its descendants).

DHA used to protect against sudden cardiac death in adults

A more careful analysis would tend to give DHA priority in the targeted prevention of sudden death syndrome, which is completely independent of cholesterol blood levels and accounted for 63.4% of cardiac disease deaths that occurred in the US during 1999. Sudden death is a cardio-respiratory arrest produced by an irregularity in the cardiac rhythm (malign ventricular arrhythmia of the ventricular tachycardia or ventricular fibrillation variety). This type of complication may occur at any time during a benign (angina pectoris) or malign (infarction) cardiac crisis. Even if its mechanism is different from the one which accounts for sudden infant death, researchers believe that these two complications are actually exacerbated by the deficiencies in omega-3 which characterize populations in the west. Harvard researchers recently demonstrated (FATS study) that a daily supplement of about 1.7g of EPA+DHA could reduce by about 40 % the risk of recurrence of malign arrhythmias among patients carrying an implantable defibrillator (ICD).

Current consensus is that we should consume at least two grams of ALA per day to obtain significant protection.
However, as in the case of EPA+DHA, higher doses will probably have greater effect, and no secondary effects need be feared if the doses are increased.

When the data go against the current

Even somewhat negative studies - those which give little a priori credence to the theory of omega-3s - have still produced arguments in support of it.

Take the study, for example, conducted among American doctors - *Physicians' Health Study*. This study showed that not only were consumers of fish not protected, but their risk actually went up. In hindsight, in fact, it appeared that these doctors had as a group accepted the idea that fish consumption protected against cardiovascular diseases and, among these doctors, it was those with the highest risk (who had in general already had a cardiac crisis) who consumed the most fish in the (justified) hope of protecting themselves from a recurrence. Thus, the increased risk was partly offset by consumption of fish among these doctors at high risk; but clearly these high-risk consumers (of fish) had totally slanted the research and caused the protective effect (the decreased risk), which was anticipated in the population as a whole, to "artificially" disappear.

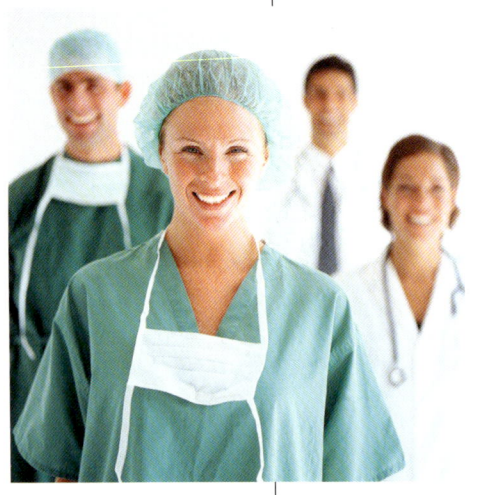

Epidemiological techniques have their limits

These studies, although very sophisticated, remain observation studies which suggest, but do not demonstrate, that omega-3s have a protective effect. In actual fact, other associated factors (preconceptions) can escape the attention of researchers. This is why the credibility of these studies depends on confirmation by randomized clinical trials conducted in proper technical conditions.

Alpha-Linolenic Acid Deficiency in the U.S.

In the US, average current consumption is about 1/2 to 2/3 what is recommended by expert committees. However, amongst the population there are numerous 'at risk' or fragile groups (young and very young, old and very old, ill, destitute, vegetarians, etc.) for which the true consumption of ALA is probably much lower. One may therefore state that, on average, the American population is deficient in ALA. In the end it is important to understand that "recommended" consumption is far from being "optimal" consumption, from the point of view of protecting oneself against certain pathologies in the long term and in different circumstances, for instance after a heart attack.

From relative deficiency to genuine scarcity

Certain nutritional habits (high consumption of omega-6) or certain treatments (anti-cholesterol medicines) can increase relative deficiencies in omega-3. They can also disrupt the metabolism of these fatty acids and produce metabolic deficiencies which, culminating in poor nutritional intake, can lead to a genuine physiological scarcity of omega-3.

CARDIOVASCULAR DISEASES: WHAT HAPPENS WHEN YOU COMPENSATE FOR OMEGA-3 DEFICIENCIES?

Data from clinical studies

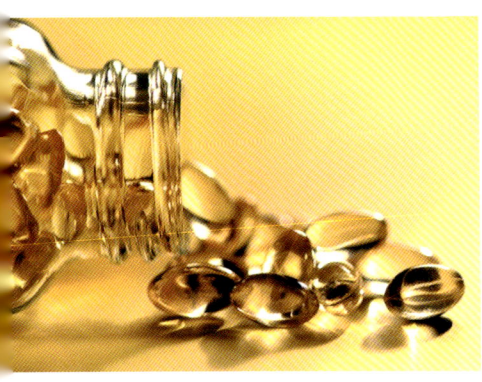

After the epidemiological studies, randomized clinical trials are the second stage of validation of the theory of omega-3s. These trials compare an experimental diet with a control diet, and participants are – like the medicines - randomly distributed in the different groups.

Better than drugs

Currently, no medicines used in cardiology, including those prescribed to lower cholesterol, have as solid a scientific profile as that of omega-3 fatty acids. None of the technically acceptable clinical omega-3 trials published to date has produced negative or even doubtful results which are capable of refuting the theory.
The truly original feature of these trials is that they were conducted at different times (between 1984 and 2002), on varied populations (British, Italian, French, Indian) with wide differences in lifestyle, and according to very different strategies. Sometimes, intervention consisted of giving very simple nutritional advice to the subjects of the trials; sometimes the nutritional advice was more complicated and the subjects were required to be carefully and closely monitored over time. At other times, concentrated fish oil capsules were prescribed.
However, all of these trials had one thing in common: the subsequent increase in

blood and tissue concentrations of omega-3 fatty acids in the experimental groups.

A universal significance

Another thing these trials have in common: the participants were, in all cases, patients who had survived a recent heart attack. They were all burdened with a serious and extremely dangerous coronary artery disease. Consequently, the lessons to be drawn from the results of these trials were of direct significance for daily clinical practice and of almost universal significance generally because patients from very different countries (in terms of ethnicity, geography and lifestyle) were included in these different trials.

The fact that benefits accrued to patients at high risk and that these benefits were reproduced elsewhere, demonstrates clearly that omega-3 fatty acids - in sufficient doses - lead to significant reduction in the risk of cardiovascular diseases or complications.

In contrast to most prevention medicines, the effect of omega-3 fatty acids on life expectancy is dramatic!

Reasons for success

The success of these trials, which was not at all expected by the many doctors whose conception of medicine is limited to drugs, can be easily explained. This was not a medical treatment intended to inhibit an enzyme, block a receptor membrane or poison such and such a cellular organelle in the hope of interrupting an injurious chain of events. It was a case of re-establishing an upset equilibrium, of correcting a deficiency and therefore of returning a disrupted physiology to normal functioning. Unlike medicines, no harmful effects were to be feared which might negate the benefits of the intervention, because the point was to reintroduce, at cellular level, nutrients indispensable to the proper functioning of cells, in other words natural substances which these cells recognize and anticipate.

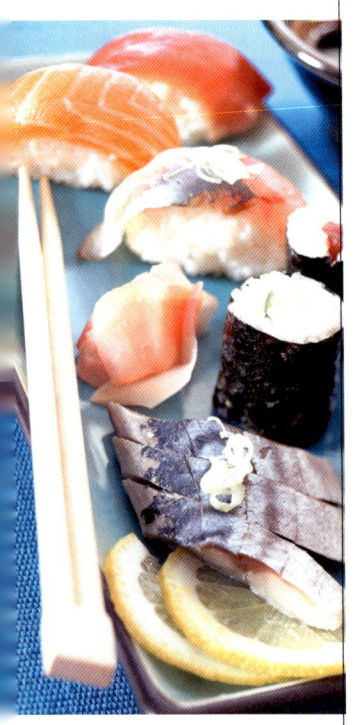

The DART study

Since 1960, the clinical arguments about the relevance of omega-3s for cardiovascular diseases have been accumulating. But it is since the DART study in 1989 that everything has really sped up.

The theory tested

Several dietary intervention trials held from the 1960s to the 1980s have suggested that a diet enriched with omega-3 fatty acids brings substantial benefits for cardiovascular prognosis.

But it was in 1989, with the DART study (*Diet And Reinfarction Trial*), that things really crystallized because, for the first time in the introduction to a randomized trial, the researchers clearly stated that they wished to test the theory that the consumption of cold water fish (rich in omega-3 fatty acids) could protect the heart.

Over 2000 patients who had survived a heart attack were recruited in Wales and randomly selected for an experimental group, where they received detailed advice on increasing their consumption of fish.

Direct effect on the heart

This dietary advice, although very simple and related to the type of fish to be consumed, the method of preparation and some general nutritional recommendations, was repeatedly given (more than eleven encounters between the investigators and the patients) during hospital consultations or visits by dieticians to patients' homes.

The following two years registered a significant decrease in global mortality (-30 %) and cardiac

CARDIOVASCULAR DISEASES: WHAT HAPPENS WHEN YOU COMPENSATE FOR OMEGA-3 DEFICIENCIES?

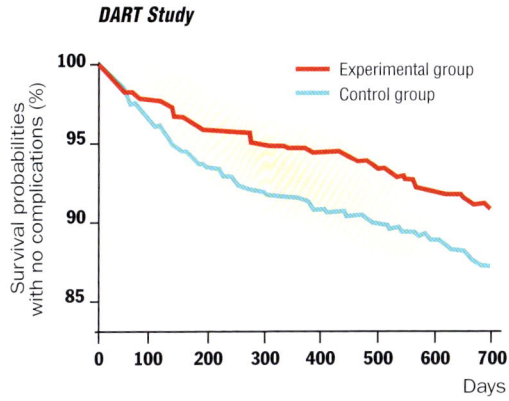

mortality (-30 %), but without any alteration in the risk of non-mortal heart attack and other cardiovascular complications.

The conclusion was as follows: the protective nutrients concerned were probably omega-3 fatty acids and this protection was generated through an effect on certain heart **rhythm disorders**, and not on the progression of artery arteriosclerosis. The significant discovery, therefore, was that this was a specifically myocardial protective effect (bearing no direct relation, in principal, to the process of artery arteriosclerosis): it was therefore possible to protect the heart itself (independently of vascular disease) and not only to counteract artery arteriosclerosis.

Lessons to be learned from the DART study

The clinical message which could be directly applied by doctors and their patients was of great significance by itself, but this trial also had a considerable impact among cardiac biologists and physiologists who launched numerous research programs to try and understand the myocardial properties (anti-arrhythmic) of omega-3 fatty acids. Since only EPA and DHA are present in significant quantities in the flesh of fatty fish consumed by the patients of the DART study, their precursor ALA excited little interest. In the end, many doctors, epidemiologists and pharmacologists, unconvinced of the nutritional theory of cardiovascular diseases, held that the DART data were impossible and were inevitably the result of chance or of some bias in the trial.

Later, they were proven wrong, but it was primarily their patients (not protected) who suffered for this lack of foresight.

The Lyon study in France

Five years after the DART study, in 1994, the results of the Lyon Diet Heart Study were published, a randomized trial aimed at testing the effect of a Mediterranean diet enriched in omega-3 fatty acids (of vegetable origin) on the risk of cardiovascular complications after a first heart attack.

Omega-3 margarine

The patients randomly selected for the experimental group were instructed on the Mediterranean diet - a simplified version - and encouraged to adopt it with their families.

The control group were required to follow the nutritional advice customarily given to cardiac patients in hospitals, in other words the diet recommended by the American Heart Association, which is described as "prudent". The patients from the control group, therefore, were recommended anything but a poor diet and they also benefited from advice relating to healthy living (smoking, exercise, etc), which is normally given to patients after a cardiac attack.

Enrichment with omega-3 was based on a different strategy to the strategy of the DART study. The patients were not required to eat more fish but rather more foods rich in ALA, essentially

A rigorous and impeccable method

After publication of the Lyon study, like the DART study, certain disgruntled people involved made it known in an underhand manner that they did not hold to the results of this trial. But many researchers, especially in the United States, considered from then on that the Lyon trial was the first trial to succeed in adequately testing the nutritional/ Mediterranean theory at a methodological level. The methods used in this study (notably the statistical analyses carried out by independent statisticians) were meticulously described in six articles in leading Anglo-Saxon scientific journals, and they did not leave themselves open to any serious criticism.

CARDIOVASCULAR DISEASES: WHAT HAPPENS WHEN YOU COMPENSATE FOR OMEGA-3 DEFICIENCIES?

rapeseed oil. To help the patients avoid butter, they and their families were recommended canola margarine for the whole duration of the trial.

Dramatic results

Over 600 patients were recruited and this cohort proved extremely reliable, in both trial groups; to such a degree that in 1998, at final analysis, the investigators had precise information on the state of health and way of life of all but four patients.

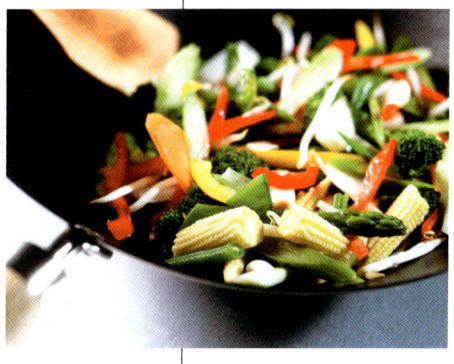

The results of the Lyon study were published in two stages (1994 and 1999) in accordance with the advice of the Scientific committee which, for obvious ethical reasons, recommended that these dramatic results be communicated to the general public as fast as possible (in other words, an intermediate analysis in advance of the final report). Dramatic, in fact, because all relevant risks (of death, of cardiac death, of new heart attacks and of all the other coronary complications) were reduced by at least 50 %, and up to 70 % for some complications.

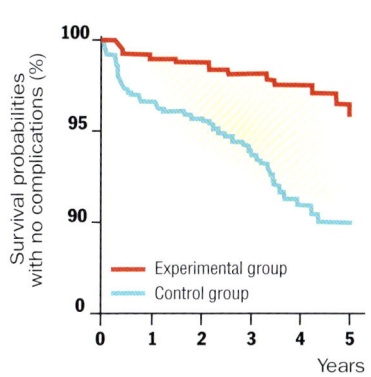

Lessons from the Lyon study

Which nutrients are responsible for the positive results of the Lyon study? In first place - the omega-3s, including alpha-linolenic acid (ALA)!

Primary cause of cardiac mortality: sudden death syndrome

One of the strong points of the Lyon study is that the researchers provided a detailed description in their report of the causes of death. This point is very important if we are to understand how a particular treatment or preventive measure acts (or fails to act). Curiously, most trials using anti-cholesterol medicines are very imprecise on these clinical aspects. In fact, the great majority of deaths of cardiac origin (60 to 75 %, depending on the populations concerned) are due to sudden cardiac death syndrome which itself, in 80 to 90 % of cases, is the consequence of a malign ventricular arrhythmia. The two main "classical" risk factors for cardiac diseases, cholesterol and high blood pressure, are poorly predictive - or not predictive at all - of sudden death. This undoubtedly explains the lack of precision of researchers in testing the medicines to reduce cholesterol and blood pressure. Since these medicines had little or no effect on sudden death syndrome, they therefore had little or no effect on cardiac mortality.

If the main objective of the trial was to test a comprehensive Mediterranean diet, the analyses conducted to find out which nutrients were responsible for the protective effect observed in the Lyon study showed that omega-3s, especially ALA and DHA, were the primary protective factors. Even if one cannot conclude that only omega-3s had a protective effect, one can say that they played a fundamental role, and that the Lyon study may be placed in the category of trials to test omega-3 fatty acids.

Secondly, the Lyon study was to be distinguished from the DART study not only in that cardiac mortality was reduced, but also because the risk of recurrence of non-mortal heart attack was also reduced. That would suggest that ALA supplementation had different clinical

CARDIOVASCULAR DISEASES: WHAT HAPPENS WHEN YOU COMPENSATE FOR OMEGA-3 DEFICIENCIES?

properties from exclusively EPA+DHA supplementation, the principal omega-3 fatty acids of fatty fish.

In actual fact, in administering ALA, the properties of both ALA and of EPA are accumulated because EPA is synthesized in our cells from ALA. Later on we will see how the situation is different for DHA. One may ask if the apparently greater clinical efficacy of ALA is due to the particular characteristics of ALA or the fact that with ALA, the protections resulting from ALA and EPA are accumulated.

AHA Science Advisory

Lyon Diet Heart Study
Benefits of a Mediterranean-Style, National Cholesterol Education Program/American Heart Association Step I Dietary Pattern on Cardiovascular Disease

Penny Kris-Etherton, PhD, RD; Robert H. Eckel, MD; Barbara V. Howard, PhD; Sachiko St. Jeor, PhD, RD; Terry L. Bazzarre, PhD; for the Nutrition Committee, Population Science Committee, and Clinical Science Committee of the American Heart Association

These extraordinary similarities (and also these differences) between the DART and Lyon studies will be confirmed by other studies, notably the big GISSI study (*page 48*).

Headline of an article of the American Heart Association recommending the experimental diet proposed by the Lyon study for cardiovascular protection or prevention of cardiovascular disease

Impact as wide as the United States and Australia

We will conclude our comments on the Lyon study by reminding any still-skeptical readers that in 2001, the *American Heart Association*, following many editorials and much commentary on this study (including in the general press), has finally updated its "official nutritional recommendations". These new recommendations, it must be said, are suspiciously like the experimental "Mediterranean" diet tested in the Lyon study!

The GISSI study

The GISSI study (acronym for "Italian group for the study of survival post infarction"), published in 1999 and in 2002, has provided crucial information on long-chain omega-3, which significantly complements the information achieved through the DART and the Lyon studies.

The GISSI strategy was different from that of the DART and the Lyon studies because it was no longer a case altering the diet of patients who had survived a heart attack, but of selecting them at random to receive (or not) concentrated fish oil capsules, each one containing about 1 g of EPA+DHA.

It was therefore a trial aimed at testing the specific effects of the EPA+DHA association. More than 11,000 patients were recruited by over 270 cardiologists all over Italy. The context was therefore very real (the researchers were not selecting the patients), and the patients who were subject to random selection were of all kinds. It was a trial occurring in "real conditions" representing everyday medicine, and consequently the lessons are immediately applicable to real life by all doctors for all patients.

After a post-trial follow-up of three and a half years, comprehensive analyses of the results revealed that the omega-3s had reduced mortality

Also vitamin E

GISSI researchers actually established four groups by random selection to test, among other things, a vitamin E tablet: control group, omega-3 group, vitamin E group and vitamin E + omega-3 group. Although the vitamin E group showed less significant results than the groups with omega-3s, some protection could still be detected, which suggests that in certain conditions vitamin E supplement might be beneficial. In contrast to the omega-3s, for which other trials are available demonstrating their beneficial effects (the DART and Lyon studies, for instance), the other publications relating to vitamin E are very contradictory and haven't enabled the encouraging data from GISSI to be confirmed.

CARDIOVASCULAR DISEASES: WHAT HAPPENS WHEN YOU COMPENSATE FOR OMEGA-3 DEFICIENCIES?

by 20 %, specific cardiac mortality by 30 % and above all sudden death (due to ventricular rhythm disorders) by 45 %.

On the other hand, the risk of recurrence of non-mortal cardiac crisis had not altered, just as in the DART study. Such concordances are an extraordinary validation of the theory of omega-3s.

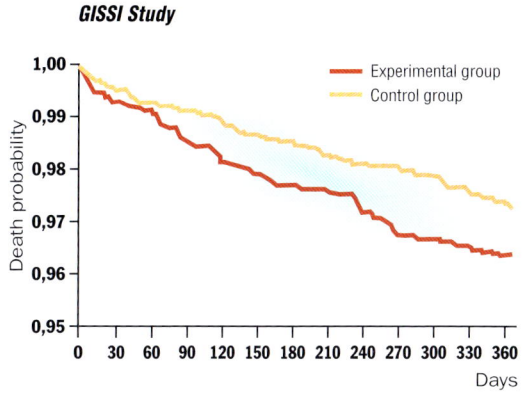

GISSI Study

Doubt is no longer permitted!

These results were comprehensively super-imposable on those of the DART study, and confirmed the results of the Lyon study, which had the big advantage of finally putting the doubters to rest.

On the biological level, doubt was no longer permitted: Omega-3s had effectively prevented a large number of ventricular arrhythmias and sudden deaths from taking place. Since publication of the DART study, many teams of biologists and physiologists had reached the same conclusions. However, contrary to the Lyon study, no effect was registered on non-mortal recurrences (as with the DART study), and therefore probably none either on the progression of arterial disease.

This was obviously only true for the test doses administered (0.8 g per day of EPA+DHA) which were modest doses, corresponding to an intake of about two portions of fatty fish (salmon, mackerel, sardine) per week.

The doses were **nutritional** and **not pharmacological.**

In other words, although the omega-3s came in the form of capsules, this investigation remained within the confines of habitual nutrition. It is probable that the protective effect observed on the whole of the population tested was the result of correcting the chronic deficiency in omega-3s among a certain number of patients.

The advent of the Mediterranean diet

The GISSI study showed that an EPA+DHA supplement of low dose was not equivalent to an ALA supplement like the one used in the Lyon study, where the reduction in risks included a reduction in the risk of non-mortal recurrence.

All the GISSI patients were advised (before randomization) to follow a Mediterranean diet (olive oil, fresh fruits and vegetables, cereals) and the researchers assessed whether, at the end of the trial, those who had most closely observed this advice had a better prognosis.
They found that those who had followed the better Mediterranean diet had seen **their risk of death reduce by close to 50%**, compared with those who had discarded it, whatever the group (omega-3, vitamin E, the two together or neither) and whatever the other risk factors that applied (age, smoking, cholesterol, weight, blood pressure, diabetes).

The GISSI study, as well as confirming the results of the DART study, therefore also supported the results of the Lyon study and the concept of a Mediterranean

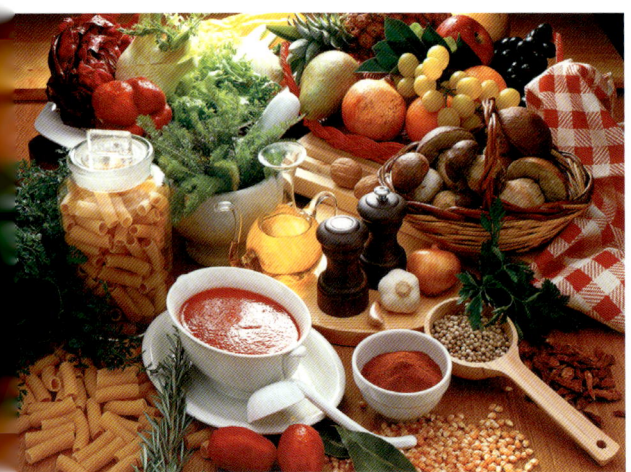

diet in general. For these reasons, the GISSI study was a turning-point in the evolution of ideas about the role of nutrition in cardiovascular diseases. Many doctors and researchers suddenly understood that the "heart and nutrition" issue was not primarily a question of cholesterol; on the contrary, they realized that the question of cholesterol (systematically promoted by the pharmacological industry) actually helped to mask the real physiopathological issues and divert the attention of doctors away from the crucial issue of cardiovascular disease prevention. In actual fact, in the DART study, the Lyon study and the GISSI study, protected patients actually had the same cholesterol levels as patients who had a recurrence or who died.

After the Lyon study and the American-Greek epidemiological study described below, the GISSI study showed how difficult it was going to be to refute the theory that dietary habits were the principal cause of cardiovascular diseases.

Confirmation from Greece

In June 2003, Antonia Trichopoulou and her colleagues from the universities of Athens and of Harvard (Boston) published the results of an epidemiological study conducted in Greece on over 22,000 adults observed over almost four years. At the start of the study, the researchers had assessed the dietary habits of each individual and set up a score allowing each of them to be classified into categories approximating to what is considered to be the traditional Mediterranean diet in contemporary Greece.

A difference of barely two units from the adherence score to this traditional diet is associated with considerable differences in the risk of dying whether from a form of cancer (a difference of 24 %) or from a heart attack (33 %).

These dramatic results thus confirmed the nutritional theory of cardiovascular diseases (and of cancers) and confirmed that if optimal health is to be the primary objective, then the fundamentals of the Mediterranean diet should be the basis of every dietary prevention strategy.

Everything depends on the nutritional context

The GISSI study showed that in the context of a Mediterranean diet, by definition rich in monounsaturated fatty acids (above all oleic acid) and in natural antioxidants (but poor in saturated fatty acids and omega-6 polyunsaturated fatty acids), one can easily see the benefits of very long-chain omega-3s, at a dose of 0.8 g per day. To put it another way, it is uncertain whether identical benefits would have been found in a different nutritional context (for instance with a high intake of polyunsaturated fats) or at higher doses (such as those recommended for treatment of inflammatory pathologies).

New evidence

The results of the *Indian Heart Trial* in 1992 and especially of the *Indo-Mediterranean Diet Trial* in 2002 support the idea that omega-3s are protective in effect and also that the best protection is probably provided through a proper combination of different series of fatty acids.

Mustard and soybean oils

No researcher would dare quibble with the well-founded wisdom of a diet low in saturated fats (essentially of animal origin) in western countries. In relation to the other fatty acids (notably omega-6 polyunsaturates and monounsaturates), a broad consensus does not yet exist despite publication of the trials, and especially the Lyon study.

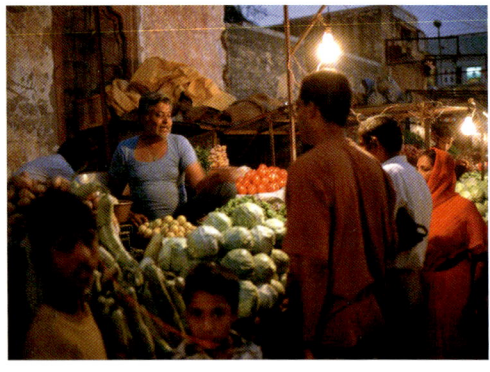

In the Indo-Mediterranean trial, more than 1000 patients who survived a recent heart attack were randomly selected to observe either a prudent post-heart attack diet generally recommended by cardiologists (control group), or a vegetarian-style diet enriched with omega-3 of vegetable origin. This experimental diet was largely inspired by the Lyon study, except that because the researchers had neither olive nor canola oil at their disposal, they recommended that their patients use soybean oil and mustard oil, two oils relatively rich in ALA and traditionally used in India. The rest of the diet closely followed the dietary recommendations used in the Lyon study (abundance of fresh and dried fruit and vegetables and low consumption of animal products).

The results were very positive, with a reduction in the frequency of non-mortal recurrences and also a reduction of sudden deaths. Most commentators hailed this study as a brilliant new confirmation of the theory celebrating the benefits of the Mediterranean diet on the one hand, and of omega-3s on the other. It also

CARDIOVASCULAR DISEASES: WHAT HAPPENS WHEN YOU COMPENSATE FOR OMEGA-3 DEFICIENCIES?

demonstrated that the nutritional theory of cardiovascular diseases stood up to criticism, even in geographic and social contexts different from the West. These data gave this theory a universal status.

Could have done better!

In actual fact, a careful reading of the data tells us that the results were not in actual fact ideal. The risk of new mortal heart attacks (through a mechanism other than sudden death) and especially the total mortality risk level were not, in fact, significantly reduced in this trial, even if the trend was in the right direction. Moreover, if consumption of omega-3 had effectively increased, that of omega-6 had not decreased and that of oleic acid remained low - two features which made this diet diverge noticeably from the Mediterranean diet in general and from the diet tested in the Lyon study in particular. This can be explained by the oils used in this trial (soy and mustard) which are too rich in omega-6.

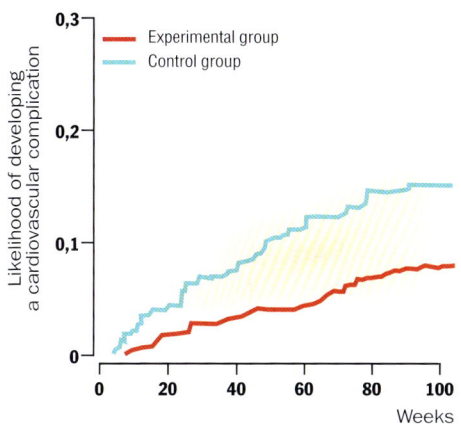

Indo-Mediterranean Study

A balance to be found

It appears that optimum benefit can be obtained from omega-3s only in the context of a Mediterranean diet with a low consumption of omega-6 fatty acids and a high consumption of oleic acid. Why is this equilibrium between the different families of fatty acids so important?
- Excessive quantities of omega-6 *(read page 19)* interfere with omega-3s, which henceforth are prevented from realizing their full protective capacity.
- One may equally suppose that since they are sensitive to oxidative stress, omega-3s are relatively "protected" in the presence of oleic acid (which is a proper antioxidant), while they are all the more "subject to attack" in the presence of significant quantities of omega-6 which are themselves pro-oxidants.

CARDIOVASCULAR DISEASES: HOW DO OMEGA-3s PROTECT THE HEART?

Three protective effects

As convincing as they are, the clinical trials and epidemiological studies rarely offer biological explanations. Obviously, scientists are not easily convinced of a phenomenon if they do not understand the mechanisms operating behind the observed effect.

The anti-arrhythmic effects of omega-3 confirmed

A German group has demonstrated an unusually high level of prevention of ventricular arrhythmias, brought on voluntarily by doctors using omega-3 solutions by intravenous drip, with almost immediate protective effect *(Lancet 2004)*.

The Alexander Leaf group in Boston reported the results of the FATS study, a double-blind trial for patients carrying an implantable defibrillator owing to a history of sudden death or equivalent syndrome. With just 1.7 g of EPA+DHA, they report a reduction of 40 % in the risk of recurrence.

Three mechanisms may be described, which explain how very long-chain omega-3 fatty acids (EPA and DHA) protect the heart.

An effect on ion channels

The team of Alexander Leaf in Boston may be credited with having discovered the effects of omega-3 fatty acids on the ion channels of cardiac cells, and therefore on the electrical activity of these cells. This electrical activity is essential for coordination of the mechanical activity of the heart *(see box)*. Omega-3s, by modulating the activity of some ion channels, stabilize the electrical activity of the cells (they are less excitable). This "stabilizing" effect is particularly important during an ischemic attack, or when the heart is deprived of oxygen due to occlusion of the artery. This effect prevents diffusion in the tissue of chaotic electrical activity (ventricular fibrillation) which normally leads to cardiac arrest.

An effect on the vegetative nervous system

A diet enriched in omega-3 has profound consequences for the nerves of the vegetative nervous system (sympathetic and parasympathetic system) which controls the electrical activity of the heart and especially the variability of cardiac rhythm. Cardiac variability refers to the propensity of the heart to vary in frequency in response to events (for instance effort or emotion). The higher the instantaneous variability of cardiac rhythm, the lower is the risk of ventricular fibrillation.

Danish researchers have demonstrated that the variability of cardiac rhythm strongly depends on omega-3 concentration in the heart and blood. They have even demonstrated, in a double-blind trial, that increasing one's intake of omega-3 will produce a very marked increase in cardiac variability, and therefore a reduction of the risk of malign ventricular arrhythmia.

"Vaccination" against cardiac crisis

The cardiac muscle is capable of developing its own defenses to withstand the effects of oxygen deprivation resulting from occlusion of the coronary artery: if the brief occlusion of a coronary artery (1 or 2 minutes) is induced several times, prior to a longer occlusion (30 to 60 minutes) which inevitably provokes cellular destruction (heart attack), the mass of necrotized tissue observed is at least **two times smaller** than in the absence of these brief prior occlusions. This is a kind of vaccination effect against the damage which a cardiac crisis is capable of inflicting on the heart muscle. Numerous teams have sought to understand the precise **preconditioning** mechanism involved and to perfect (without success so far) new molecules susceptible of imitating it, in the hope of developing new medicines from them. In actual fact, only two preventive interventions, both dietary, have enabled the ischemic preconditioning to be reproduced: **moderate alcohol consumption** and - in particular - **consumption of omega-3 fatty acids!**

And alpha-linolenic acid?

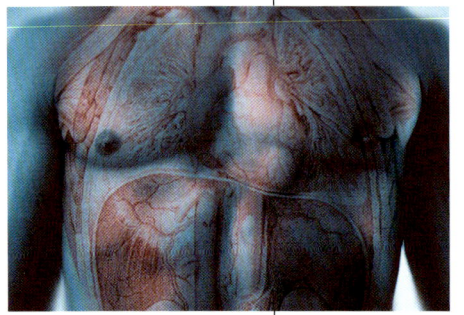

The three mechanisms described above are probably the most important ones in explaining the protective effects on the heart of EPA and DHA. But how does alpha-linolenic acid (ALA) act?

ALA as the precursor to EPA

Since EPA has cardio-protective effects, it might be thought that its direct precursor (ALA) had potentially the same effects. However, it is difficult to account for the protective effects of EPA and DHA, and the synthesis of DHA from EPA remains uncertain in many individuals, especially at extreme ages of life. In other words, ALA is a good precursor to EPA but not to DHA; significant intake of ALA translates in general (and notably in the Lyon study) into an increase in concentrations of EPA but not of DHA. That said, we still know very little about the specific metabolism of omega-3s in each organ. What is really happening in the heart or brain of human beings? At the present state of knowledge, no one knows.

A direct effect on the arteries

In the clinical trials, it cannot be denied that ALA supplementation brought benefits beyond those observed with EPA+DHA supplementation. For example: a significant reduction of the risk of non-mortal recurrence, which has an impact on the progression of vascular arteriosclerosis independently of the prevention of complications relating to the heart muscle, such as sudden death.

This arterial effect is confirmed by an epidemiological study which had correlated the thickness of the carotid artery walls (by sophisticated ultrasound equipment) with intake of ALA. The more ALA one consumes, the less the carotid artery wall is subject to thickening.

An uncertain effect on ischemia

In certain experimental models (notably those relating to malign arrhythmias and sudden death syndrome), the perfusion of ALA has had similar effects to those of EPA or DHA. However, it is known that the quantity of ALA available in cardiac membranes (susceptible of being liberated by ischemic stress in order to exercise its anti-arrhythmic potential) is very low, which considerably weakens the hypothesis that ALA plays an important role during an acute ischemia.

Finally, although this is certainly not the most important protective mechanism in clinical medicine, it is probably because it interacts in the metabolism of omega-3 and omega-6 essential fatty acids that ALA exercises its protective effect at the doses tested in the clinical trials.

Clearly, not only does ALA not act like EPA, but it also acts very like an anti-omega-6.

EPA is not DHA

Is it legitimate to differentiate between the biological effects of EPA and DHA? Even if neuropsychiatry would lead one to believe that EPA and DHA have particular characteristics *(read page 105)*, cardiologists do not generally distinguish between them. In fact, it even seems that DHA may have more specifically cardiological properties than EPA. This would not be surprising in view of their respective concentrations in tissues, notably for example in the cardiac mitochondria membranes which contain a significantly higher quantity of DHA than EPA.

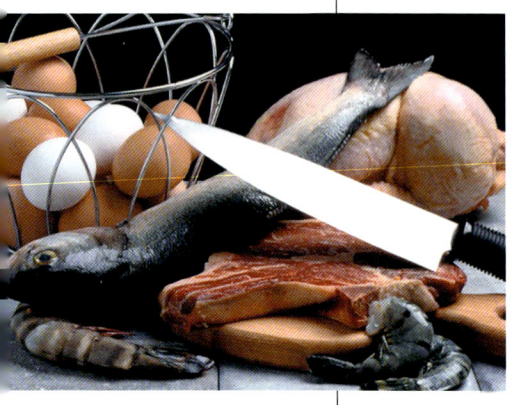

Open competition between omega-3 and omega-6

Not only is ALA the precursor to EPA but it is also the competitor of linoleic acid (the principal source of omega-6 in our food) for the synthesis of the latter's descendents, especially arachidonic acid (AA), the main mediator of inflammation, notably vascular inflammation.

Healthy competition

AA, from the Omega-6 family, is the precursor of many substances which encourage inflammation, vessel constriction, formation of clots and atheroma plaques in the arteries. There is no doubt that the decline in the synthesis of these substances through the simple reduction in AA (result of competition between ALA and linoleic acid and reducing consumption of foods containing AA such as meat, eggs, poultry) has a protective effect on the arteries. EPA may also be in competition with AA for the synthesis of its descendants, and it is recognized to possess real anti-inflammatory and antithrombotic properties.

Do omega-3s carry the risk of hemorrhage?

This problem is somewhat "theoretical" because the specific protective effect on the cardiac muscle described in previous pages was obtained through low dietary intake (around 1 g per day of EPA+DHA or 2 g of ALA, doses with little significant effect on coagulation and platelets). This suggests that anti-thrombotic mechanisms, while not completely absent at these low doses, probably play a minor role with many patients. That said, at doses of at least 3 g per day, some laboratories have observed minor effects on coagulant factors, such as fibrinogen, and on functional parameters (thrombin generation) without knowing the clinical importance (favorable or harmful) of these small variations.

Because a high consumption of ALA has the double advantage of increasing EPA concentrations and reducing AA cells, we have an inkling of how ALA may prove to be a powerful agent for vascular protection.

Omega-3s inhibit platelets

Therefore they potentially reduce the risk of thrombosis (blood clots). This action on the blood platelets is again the result of competition with omega-6s. The overall effect on the risk of thrombosis is therefore the consequence of a new equilibrium between the anti-platelet effect and the way in which omega-3s act to maintain the capacity of the vascular endothelium to generate prostacycline, an anti-platelet and vasodilator prostaglandin.

By their effect on the metabolism of triglycerides, omega-3 fatty acids could also interfere with the coagulation pathways, notably at factor VII level.

It is known that high consumption of omega-3 results in increased bleeding time comparable to the effect of aspirin. This has actually been observed among Eskimos, who consume up to 7-10 g of omega-3 per day. For this reason, some scientists recommend that one should not combine anticoagulant treatments with high doses of omega-3 due to the potential risk of hemorrhage, for instance during a surgical operation.

The benefits of competition

The team of James Dwyer at the University of Southern California has shown, in an article in the *New England Journal of Medicine* published in 2004, that competition between EPA and AA at the level of the 5-lipoxygenase* enzyme is all the more alive because individuals are carriers of a variant of the 5-lipoxygenase gene promoter. Certainly, only 6 % of the 470 subjects studied were carriers of this genetic feature in this study, but this constituted a real handicap in terms of vascular pathology especially if their intake of AA was significant. However, a high consumption of EPA tended to eliminate this genetically determined handicap.

The 5-lipoxygenase enzyme is an enzyme which regulates the synthesis of pro-inflammatory substances called leucotrienes which are implicated especially in asthma.

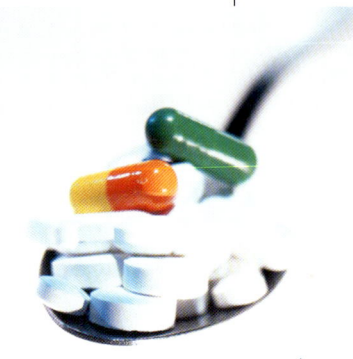

Other potential protective mechanisms

Beyond their specific effects on the cardiac muscle, omega-3 fatty acids have a beneficial effect on other "classic" risk factors such as the triglycerides or blood pressure.

Omega-3s reduce triglycerides

The more omega-3 we consume and the more omega-3 we have in our tissues, the less we come up against the anomaly of the triglycerides. However, to obtain a clinically significant reduction of these lipids in the blood, we must consume several grams of omega-3 per day, and no clinical trial testing high doses of omega-3 has yet shown that reducing triglycerides will have a significant protective effect on the heart.

Omega-3s reduce blood pressure

At high doses (4 to 8 g per day), omega-3s reduce blood pressure and cardiac rate, especially for subjects with high blood pressure or obesity, or those with an elevated level of blood lipids. Some researchers believe that omega-3s amplify the effect of high blood pressure medicines. These data are not surprising when one bears in mind the importance of nutrition in high blood pressure. This

An unfortunate fascination for drugs in high blood pressure

Salt in food but also potassium, magnesium and calcium all play a role in the activation and continuation of high blood pressure. An excellent American study known as the DASH study has shown that a diet rich in fruit and vegetables (source of potassium and magnesium), poor in saturated fats and in sodium but also including skimmed milk products (source of calcium) was as effective as a medicine (in monotherapy) to reduce blood pressure.

effect is associated with a relaxant effect on the arteries and appears almost exclusively the result of DHA, without any noticeable effect from EPA. There are no data on ALA.

Elevated triglycerides, a health risk?

The higher the level of triglycerides, the higher the apparent increase in cardiovascular risk. This increased risk is minimal as long as the increase in the level of triglycerides is controlled. However, triglycerides are a good marker of risk associated with metabolic syndromes (*see page 90*).

What about high doses?

Can one safely take high doses of omega-3 **(over 3 g per day of EPA+DHA)**? Caution is required, because these fatty acids are very sensitive to oxidation and we cannot be sure that they are totally harmless. If EPA+DHA doses of several grams are used, then one's intake of omega-6 must be lowered (proportionately) at the same time, so that the total intake of polyunsaturates (omega-3 and omega-6) remains low overall. One must also take care to ensure that one's intake of natural antioxidants is in proportion to the omega-3s. A high-dose supplementation of omega-3 should ideally be associated with a traditional Mediterranean diet (poor in saturated and polyunsaturated fatty acids, rich in monounsaturates and natural antioxidants) such as the diet used for the Lyon and GISSI studies. As a precautionary measure, we advise that a high- or very high-dose supplement should be of short duration and after an initial treatment, a more moderate dose should be taken.

PREVENT CANCER WITH OMEGA-3s

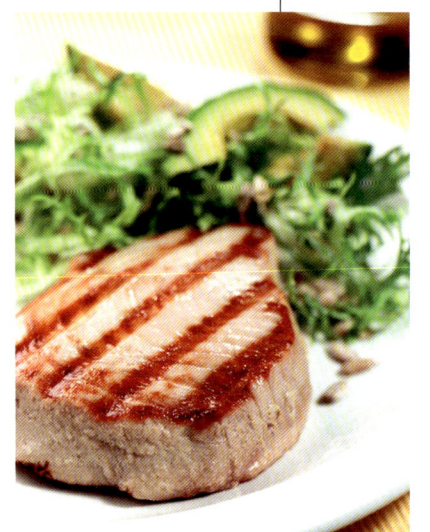

Populations which consume a lot of omega-3 (Japanese, Mediterranean populations which have maintained their traditional dietary customs) have a clearly reduced risk of cancer compared with other populations, especially in the west.

There is not "one" cancer!

Fewer data exist on the links between omega-3 and cancer (and between dietary factors and cancers in general) than on cardiovascular diseases in general. However, the data that do exist suggest that omega-3s can help reduce the cancer risk. One of the problems for researchers stems from the fact that each type of cancer is a disease in itself with its own specific causes and treatments. The evidence shows that throat cancer, for instance, does not respond to the same determining factors as breast or prostate cancer.

Still, there is no doubt that suitable **omega-3 intake contributes to lowering the risk of cancer, whereas high omega-6 consumption increases this risk,** because omega-3s are the constituents of all cell membranes, and due to their anti-proliferation and anti-dissemination properties.

Must one wait for irrefutable "proof" before action is taken?

The principal carcinogenic factor is the time factor: on the one hand the duration of exposure to carcinogenic factors (for instance smoking), and on the other the time required for the development of a clinically detectable tumor. In contrast with cardiovascular illnesses, there are no cataclysmic events in cancer resulting in death in a matter of minutes; instead we are dealing with a slow, chronic disease. In the same way, there is no distinction between primary and secondary prevention (prevention of recurrence), because again the time factor has been an obstacle to researchers. This means that as we confront the epidemic of cancer now attacking western populations, it would be absurd to make the elaboration of a prevention strategy depend on irrefutable proof (which possibly will never exist).

Therefore the precautionary principle needs to be rigorously applied, particularly since a dietary anti-cancer strategy can be practically superimposed over the prevention strategy for cardiovascular diseases, since there are no harmful effects to be feared and, above all, since we have nothing to lose!

Epidemiology: inconclusive

Epidemiological cancer studies are very inconclusive, the main problem again being one of "time". In actual fact, if one examines the correspondences between a cancer and a nutritional factor, once the cancer is diagnosed (a so-called "case control" study), it is not safe to draw conclusions about causality. Perhaps it is the cancer which has produced the nutritional factors and not the other way round.

If the dietary habits of the subjects concerned are studied very early in life (when one may be certain that they do not yet have cancer), because one is waiting several decades for cancers to make their appearance (prospective study), it is probable that many other factors, including dietary factors, will have modified during this long time period. From that moment on, to what can we credibly attribute the onset of these cancers?

To meet these difficulties, the researchers recruited very large cohorts in the hope (misguided), that quantity might make up for the absence of quality. They also used complicated mathematical models ("meta-analyses" for example) to enable them to collate the results of several studies and produce one large study out of them. Unfortunately these statistics were no substitute for quality data.

Breast cancer

The frequency of breast cancer varies a lot from one geographical region to another, and hormonal or genetic factors only in part explain this variability.

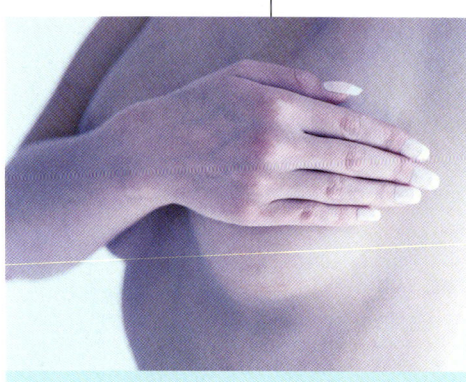

Chemotherapy + omega-3

To treat cancers which have already been diagnosed, some researchers seek to combine chemotherapy and dietary modifications with dietary enrichment by omega-3. Despite the absence of conclusive proof, we advise doctors in charge of patients undergoing chemotherapy to encourage them to increase their consumption of omega-3. It has been clearly demonstrated that they could delay the onset of some systemic inflammatory complications (malnutrition, cachexia) which are relatively independent of the primitive tumor but very negative for the overall prognosis.

The dietary factors involved

During recent decades, there has been an extraordinary increase in the frequency of breast cancers, an increase which not even the best diagnostic methods can easily explain. Here again, the nutritional factor appears as the most plausible explanation. The epidemiological data are fairly clear: for example, the more fish one eats, the lower the risk of developing breast cancer. Another example: a positive correlation is apparent between consumption of oils rich in omega-6 and the risk of breast cancer.

Another way of proceeding is to evaluate the direct consumption of omega-3 fatty acids (nutrients rather than food) or to use biomarkers (omega-3 concentration in blood, circulating cells or in the breast adipose tissue). In this way too, an inverse correlation may be observed between cancer risk and omega-3s and again, a positive correlation with omega-6s. What appears significant is the **omega-6/omega-3 balance,** rather than the individual intake of each fatty acid.

Linoleic acid suspected

A team of researchers under Philippe Bougnoux in Tours, France, distinguished itself by its study into the lipid factors potentially involved in breast cancers. Research in experimental biology (mammary cancer induced in living animals or in human cancer cell cultures) is going in the same direction, with omega-3s showing an inhibitory effect on the proliferation of cancer cells. However this effect depends partly on omega-6s being present in the cell culture milieu or in the diet of the animal.

> ### The game is worth the candle!
> We acknowledge that our arguments in relation to omega-3 acids, omega-6 acids and breast cancers are far from being as solid as those for cardiovascular diseases. The main reason for this is the absence of randomized trials and the methodological problems associated with the published epidemiological studies. In the absence of clinical trials, the observational data and the experimental data must be carefully combined. So it is no exaggeration to say that if we are to prevent cancer, a proper balance must prevail between the families of essential fatty acids. Although absolute certainty is still lacking, the wager is worth the effort because no harmful effects need be feared from this re-balancing of the omega-3/omega-6 relation and because, at the same time, positive protective effects will accrue for cardiovascular diseases.

Research on the spread of tumors also indicates that omega-6 fatty acids, especially linoleic acid, are the preferred food of migrant tumor cells.

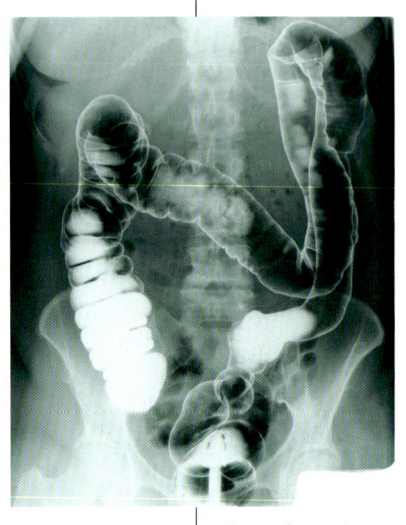

Colon and rectal cancers

These cancers are among the most frequent in the west and over 90 % of the risk can probably be attributed to dietary factors.

What are these dietary factors?

The total quantity of fats on the one hand (enabling factor) and of fibers on the other hand (inhibiting factor) are a matter of consensus among researchers. In the same way, meat consumption tends to favor colon cancer while consumption of fish should have the opposite effect.

But this information is obtained from epidemiological observation studies, and to date no causal relation has been proven. For this reason, intervention trials need to be organized, with random selection. Numerous difficulties, especially financial (lack of sponsors) but also ethical, have prevented such research from being carried out. So we are in the same situation as with breast cancer: we live in anticipation! Moreover, studies on cancer of the colon and rectum which use biomarkers (potentially more reliable studies than those which assess dietary consumption), are less definitive than those relating to breast cancer.

Omega-6 and omega-3 duality

On the other hand, there are some randomized studies on fish oils which test not the effect on the cancer risk itself but the effect on the "intermediate" markers of the risk, for example epithelial cell proliferation measured in the rectum of patients with a family history of digestive cancer. These trials generally reveal the inhibitive (and therefore protective) effect of omega-3s on this abnormal cellular proliferation which, in principle, precedes the appearance of cancers.

In some experimental models, diets enriched by corn oil (rich in omega-6) tend to accelerate the development of tumors while those enriched by fish oil (rich in omega-3) have the opposite effect. So we come back to the problem of the balance between omega-6 and omega-3. This points towards other studies which use agents (for example aspirin) to block the metabolism of arachidonic acid in humans and which have demonstrated an inhibitive effect both on the development of intestinal polyps (onto which cancerous tumors often become grafted) and on the colon cancers themselves.

The limits of animal experimentation!

One should be careful about extrapolating from animals to humans because the experimental models remain somewhat remote from the clinical reality and because most animals used in the laboratories are not sensitive to tumoral pathologies in the same way as humans are. On the other hand, research on the environmental causes of cancers among human beings is meeting almost insurmountable difficulties. Must we wait for irrefutable proof before we can take action on the issue of our health? At the risk of repeating ourselves, we believe that it is a mistake to patiently await the emergence of scientific "evidence" (which may never arise, given the difficulty in obtaining it in the first place) and that we must from this moment on rigorously apply the precautionary principle to these pathologies, even if this happens to conflict with the interests of certain agribusiness tycoons.

From Los Angeles to Lyon: the clinical studies

To date there has been no randomized trial to test a theory concerning omega-3 fatty acids and cancers. However, two trials initially conceived to test a cardiac theory have had results which are relevant to cancers.

The Los Angeles study

Even if the aim was not to study the onset of cancers and even if the sample studied was not considered with this objective in mind, one can and must take advantage of the essential methodological aspect of the randomized trial, in other words the formation by random selection of two absolutely identical groups to study the effects of nutrition on cancers.

In the Los Angeles study, the patients were randomly selected to follow a diet aimed at reducing their cholesterol and involving a tripling of their intake of linoleic acid. The reduction in cholesterol was significant (around 15 %), but the reduction in frequency of cardiac attacks was not particularly significant. Most importantly, the frequency of cancers rose in a disturbing way. Because researchers were operating within the framework of a randomized trial, the only factor which could be held responsible for this was the experimental diet. This diet was excessively rich in omega-6, with a parallel and proportionate reduction in oleic acid

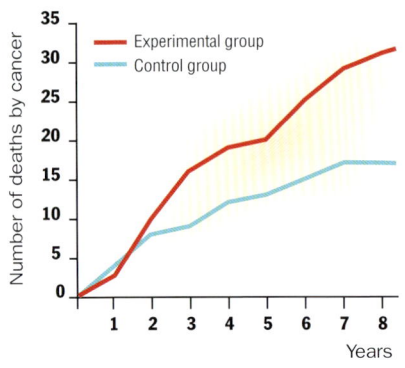

Los Angeles Study

and in the omega-3/omega-6 ratio. These clinical data are impressive and in accordance with numerous studies in experimental biology testing the pro-cancer effect of omega-6s. That said, obviously, one cannot draw any definitive conclusions about the mechanism of cancer itself.

The Lyon study

Also conceived to test a cardiac theory, this study also suggests that an inadequate diet can favor the development of various forms of cancer. In this study (already described on page 44), the objective was to compare a diet relatively rich in omega-6 and aimed at reducing cholesterol (recommended as a "prudent" diet by the *American Heart Association*) with a Mediterranean diet rich in oleic acid and in omega-3 but poor in omega-6 (therefore the precise opposite of the diet tested in Los Angeles). In this trial, it was again the patients with the highest intake of omega-6 and the lowest intake of omega-3 (the control group) who presented with the most cancers. Certainly, "one swallow doesn't make a summer" but the results of these two trials should not be ignored. They should, on the contrary, stimulate serious research in this area.

Questions which researchers must answer

In the Lyon study (as well as the Los Angeles study), several modifications of food fats and lipids could in theory explain the reduced frequency of cancers in the "Mediterranean" group of the Lyon study and in the control group of the Los Angeles study. But which of these modifications were responsible for the reduction in cancers in the Lyon study and their increase in the Los Angeles study? Another important question: given the brevity of this research (and therefore the short duration of exposure to carcinogenic factors), how does one give a biological explanation for the difference between the groups observed? So many important questions to which we must attempt a response (following section).

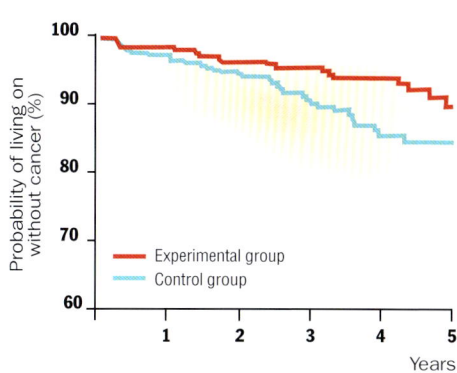

Lyon Study (cancers)

From Los Angeles to Lyon: the conclusions

Which dietary factors can explain the results of the Los Angeles and Lyon studies? What are the biological mechanisms? Here are the basic elements of a response.

Which dietary factor?

In all likelihood, the relevant issue is the overall equilibrium among the three families of fatty acids. In fact, in the experimental group of the Lyon study, less linoleic acid was used (and more oleic acid and omega-3 fatty acids), while in the Los Angeles experimental group, the use of linoleic acid tripled (with a proportionate reduction of oleic acid and of omega-3s). As a consequence, completely contrary tendencies were observed for cancers in the two experimental groups of the two trials. Other dietary factors could have played a role, especially in the Lyon study. For example, an increased intake of certain antioxidants and of fiber. Still, due to the swiftness of the clinical effect observed in both trials, we would attribute less importance to these factors. In the end it is possible that the *trans* fatty acids could have been involved, as envisaged in our article published in the Archives of Internal Medicine in 1998.

Still a question of balance

The answers to the two questions raised above suggest that what remains fundamental to the clinical surfacing of cancers (as indeed to the whole process of inflammation) are the imbalances between the omega-3 and omega-6 fatty acid families, rather than the question of increasing or decreasing the levels of a particular fatty acid.

Which biological mechanisms?

It is unlikely that these dietary differences could, in such a brief period (a few years on average), have resulted in the birth of tumors (biologists speak of an "initiation phase"). This, in actual fact, is the result of several subsequent genetic mutations which can occur only over a fairly long period, in principal several decades.

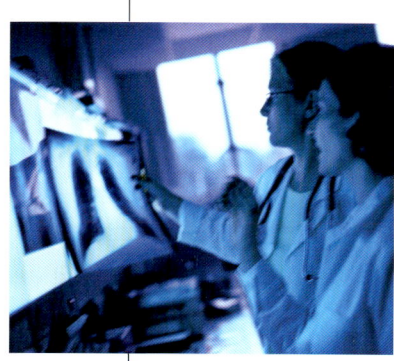

Certainly, inauspicious diets (rich in oxidant agents or in nutrients sensitive to oxidation and poor in antioxidants) can lead to the onset of tumors, but this still does not explain the rapid effects (beneficial or harmful) observed in the Los Angeles and Lyon studies.

On the other hand, these diets can act very rapidly on the clinical surfacing of tumors because this depends significantly on the inflammatory and vascular environment of the tumor.

One may suppose therefore that these diets (revealing an omega-6/omega-3 imbalance in favor of omega-6 fatty acids) have acted on tumors already present in tissue but more or less dormant. It is as if the growth and spread of the tumor around its original site was favored (even a matter of months is enough) by facilitating the generation of vasodilator and inflammatory substances (derived from arachidonic acid). The presence of significant quantities of omega-3 fatty acids could have had a contrary effect.

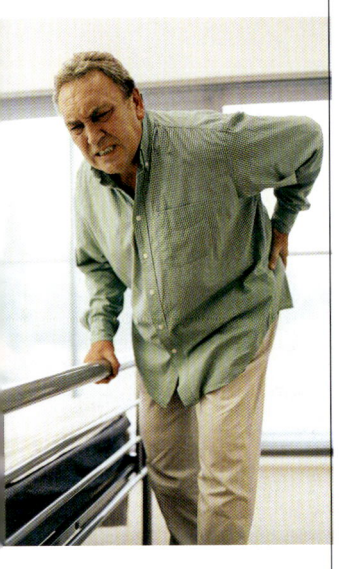

OMEGA-3s IN INFLAMMATORY DISEASES

When the immune system errs

The immune system helps us to defend ourselves against attack, whether by pollutants, toxins or microorganisms. However it can happen that it errs in its target or in the means to achieve its objective. An imbalance of omega-3 and omega-6 essential fatty acids can at least partially explain these errors.

Omega-3 deficiency suspected

Our immune defenses sometimes miss their target. They attack healthy cells in our organism and are sometimes the cause of serious illnesses. These are the auto-immune diseases, for example rheumatoid arthritis. At other times, the immune system overreacts in response to outside attack (for example in response to allergens in our environment) and we suffer the consequences in the form of diseases which are sometimes very troublesome (eczema) or dangerous (asthma).

In its battle to protect us, the immune system sets in motion an "inflammatory reaction" which also can be exaggerated in relation to the threat concerned. Anti-inflammatory treatments are often prescribed in an attempt to treat a disease or ease symptoms, even though inflammation is in reality the first necessary phase of the healing process, which has to begin by neutralizing the aggressive agents.

This poor adaptation of the immune and inflammatory response can be seen as a disease in itself and many researchers believe that a **deficiency in omega-3** (or an excess of omega-6 or, especially, both combined) contributes to these inflammatory diseases.

Omega-3s are not firemen but fireguards

In contrast to cardiovascular diseases, where doctors and researchers generally associate the manipulation of dietary omega-3 fatty acids with other dietary modifications, the approach to immune and inflammatory diseases has to date been pharmacological in nature, in other words centered exclusively on **omega-3s at elevated doses.**

This can certainly be justified where a patient is suffering from an advanced stage of the disease and can find relief through such treatment, but the effect of such a treatment is necessarily limited because **omega-3s are not anti-inflammatory medicines.** Omega-3s are primarily effective before the appearance of symptoms, when it is necessary to rebalance omega-6/omega-3 ratios and ensure that the tissue concentrations of omega-3 are adequate. In other words, "omega-3s are not fire fighters"; they should above all be used as preventive agents, not unlike fireguards.

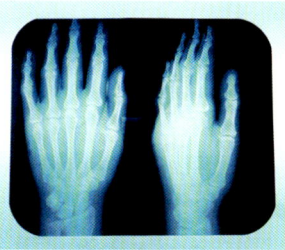

Joint diseases, inflammatory diseases

All joint diseases, including the so-called degenerative diseases linked with ageing, have an inflammatory component, which often appears very late in the development of these diseases. The dominant symptom which often reveals the existence of joint diseases and joint inflammation is articular or joint pain, which can be accompanied by a functional incapacity that is potentially very disabling.

Painful joints

Many researchers believe that arachidonic acid AA (omega-6) is largely responsible for articular inflammatory syndromes. This fatty acid is, moreover, the main target of modern treatments for joint diseases.

A mediator of joint pain

A significant mediator of joint pain is an eicosanoid called prostaglandin E2 (PGE2) which is derived directly from the principal omega-6 fatty acid in tissues, arachidonic acid (AA). AA also gives rise to other hormonal substances such as thromboxanes which stimulate the production of cytokines (TNF, interleukins) which are themselves causes of articular destruction, or again the leucotrienes which activate leucocytes which equally, through their own specific harmful action, cause articular destruction and pain.

Omega-3s impede the metabolism of AA

The main medicinal treatment for joint inflammation involves blocking the metabolism of AA (with aspirin or non-steroid anti-inflammatory medicines or hormone treatments such as cortisone or its derivatives). The therapeutic alternative more and more frequently considered involves increasing the dietary intake of omega-3 fatty acids. These compete with AA at all stages of its involvement in joint inflammation (read page 10), but without completely blocking its metabolism.

The main rival of AA is EPA, but the other omega-3s (especially ALA) can become transformed into EPA and are therefore also effective in impeding the metabolism of AA.

Some scientists believe that the main point of impact of EPA (besides its competition with AA) lies in its ability to reduce the production of cytokines which stimulate the cartilage-destroying "enzymes".

Whatever the actual mechanism, the use of omega-3s to relieve the pain from joint diseases is not new. In the past, doctors used to use fish oils to give relief to patients presenting with gout.

Complementary approaches

The pharmacological industry is currently mobilized to develop anti-cytokine medicines and make them rapidly available to doctors, the cost of which (unlike that for omega-3 fatty acids) will again be very large for the health insurance industry. However it would be foolish to oppose these two therapeutic approaches. The evidence shows that they are complementary, the idea being that omega-3 fatty acids should be used primarily as agents of prevention of acute attacks of these inflammatory diseases.

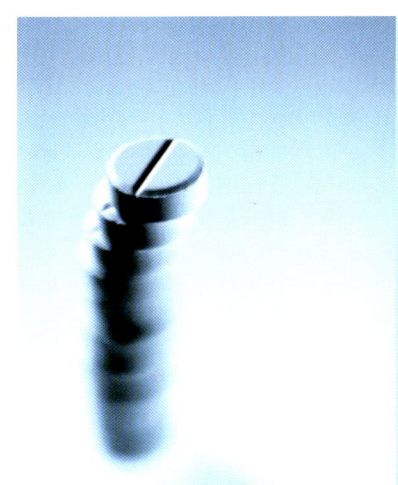

Anti-inflammatories: medicines with side effects

Anti-inflammatory medicines block the metabolism of AA by the enzyme cyclooxygenase (also called COX), the first stage for production of eicosanoids. There are several COX enzymes and one must distinguish between anti-COX-1 (the prototype being aspirin) and anti-COX-2 medicines. Unfortunately these all have side effects, sometimes harmful, such as heartburn generated by aspirin. This limits the use and dosage of these medicines for many patients. And hence the importance of complementary or alternative treatments (such as the omega-3s), which do not have side effects.

Rheumatoid arthritis

Rheumatoid arthritis is more an inflammatory than a degenerative disease, but it is very disabling. It can occur among the very young.

Omega-3s effective even in extreme conditions

Over ten randomized trials tested omega-3s in rheumatoid arthritis. The doses applied were higher (a minimum of 3 g per day of EPA+DHA) than those tested in cardiac diseases (generally less than 1 g). These doses can sometimes cause small stomach upsets which although unpleasant are not serious. There is no immediate clinical effect. Two to three months need to elapse before a definitive effect on the articular symptoms can be measured. These trials proved very encouraging and were without any dangerous side effects, even though they were conducted on patients with advanced disease and with very damaged joints – a situation obviously far from ideal when one is measuring the effectiveness of a new therapeutic approach.

The joints of Eskimos

The theory that omega-3s may be effective in treating inflammatory arthritis is also supported by the fact that populations consuming a lot of fatty fish (including the Eskimos of Greenland whose genetic profile favors joint inflammation) have fewer joint diseases than populations consuming low amounts of omega-3. Without knowing it, these populations are already applying the main principles of a *"preventive anti-inflammatory diet"*. Having said that, as the Swedish study shows *(quoted in the box opposite)*, the best dietary anti-inflammatory approach should be based on the traditional Mediterranean diet enriched in omega-3.

The ideal lies in prevention

Medical and biological logic would, however, argue that omega-3s are most effective when used for prevention or at least very early on, when the disease has just surfaced. This preventive vision contradicts modern medicine which has an essentially remedial bias. While we await new scientific studies that demonstrate the importance of early timing for this type of treatment - perhaps even before the appearance of real symptoms - nothing prevents us from starting right now to change our dietary habits: this will have the further advantage of protecting us from cardiopathies, cancers and from the other inflammatory diseases described in this chapter.

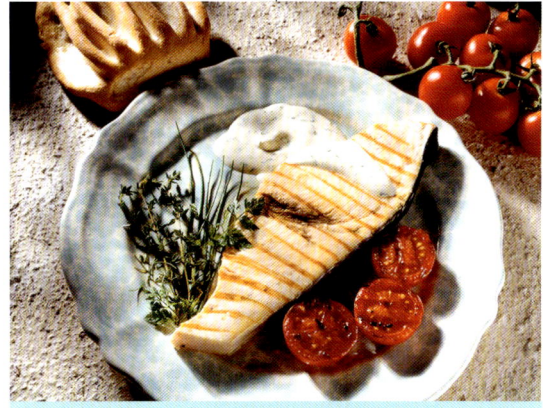

A Mediterranean diet relieves rheumatoid arthritis

Logic requires the reduction of one's intake of omega-6 and the simultaneous increase of one's intake of omega-3. Unfortunately, this type of dietary reasoning has been ignored to date by researchers in this area because they have only considered omega-3s in pharmacological form. They are probably wrong to do so, because in a recent randomized study (published in 2003), Swedish researchers tested the efficacy of a Mediterranean diet (by definition poor in omega-6 and rich in omega-3) for arthritic patients. After just a few weeks, they found a remarkable clinical improvement. Because this could not be attributed to other major elements of the Mediterranean diet such as antioxidants (due to the biological dosages required to be effective), the improvement was certainly due to the nearly ideal combination of the different families of fatty acids.

To prevent asthma

Asthma is the main respiratory inflammatory disease. Its incidence has been on the increase for several decades in the west. Children are affected earlier and earlier (occasionally from birth) and more and more seriously. Omega-3 and omega-6 essential fatty acids could have a major role to play in this epidemic.

Watch out for restrictive diets

The mother should not follow a restrictive diet aimed at reducing the number of allergens which might affect the fetus, because this could produce more general dietary deficiencies and, potentially, delayed growth such as has been observed among strict vegetarians. Care should therefore be taken when it comes to restrictive diets during pregnancy!

Fingered: Omega-3 deficiency

Some nursing infants also (or separately) present with skin diseases such as eczema which certainly respond to "allergic" processes similar to those involved in asthma. This epidemic of asthma is probably due to environmental factors amongst which (as well as exposure to new allergens such as those contained in peanuts) the "dietary fatty acid" factor appears to predominate.

The two dietary factors which emerge from recent research on infant asthma are:
1) absence of breast-feeding
2) low consumption of omega-3

Because maternal milk is in principle rich in omega-3, one may suppose that one and the same factor is involved. However, the composition of maternal milk can significantly vary depending on the dietary habits of the mother. For example, the DHA concentration in the milk of Eskimo women is much higher than that of American or European women; and the frequency of asthma among the Eskimos is very low! This is obviously not due to chance. Again, the significance of the dietary modifications which occurred during recent decades, involving reduced intake of omega-3, seems quite clear. This reduction includes reduced intake of omega-3 by nursing infants, due to the deterioration of maternal milk.

A preventive strategy

One of the most encouraging aspects of recent research on asthma in small children is that it is possible to reduce its frequency and severity by taking action prior to birth, in other words, by acting on the diet of the mother during pregnancy.

A good strategy (carrying no risk to either fetus or mother) is to increase omega-3 consumption - both vegetable and marine in origin - during pregnancy, especially in the third trimester and to continue during lactation, which should last at least four months if possible. Under these conditions, in fact, it is assumed that the maternal metabolism will properly regulate the intake of the fetus and then of the baby in accordance with its specific needs, without an excess of omega-3 occurring for the fetus (or an imbalance between omega-3s and arachidonic acid) (*see page 95*).

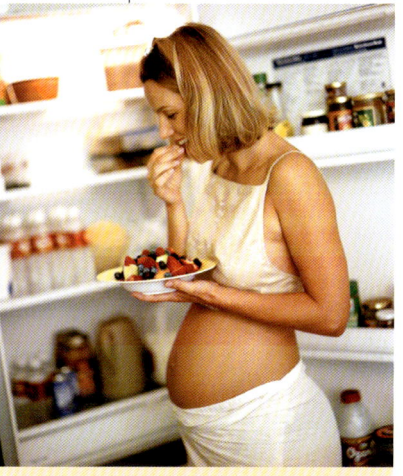

A new preventive medicine

To act on the mother's diet to prevent asthma in the infant... this transgenerational approach opens completely new perspectives in preventive medicine or in medicine full stop, because it suggests that the health of all of us, as adults too, depends partly on factors which preceded our birth, especially the dietary habits of our mothers during their pregnancy; and the same is true for pathologies other than asthma.

When asthma has taken hold

Once asthma has taken hold, a change of diet in favor of omega-3 fatty acids can produce significant improvements.

Very encouraging randomized trials

In adult asthma, the problem is difficult to analyze because most of the studies dealt with diseases which were generally quite advanced (probably involving irreversible bronchial alterations) among patients (including infants and adolescents) taking numerous medicines which in themselves were toxic (cortisones or derivatives), but which treating doctors believed were necessary to prescribe. However, certain trials involving increased intake of omega-3 were seen as very encouraging, especially among children, and a clear tendency emerged for reduction in the need for medicines - an indirect proof of the effectiveness of omega-3s in this context.

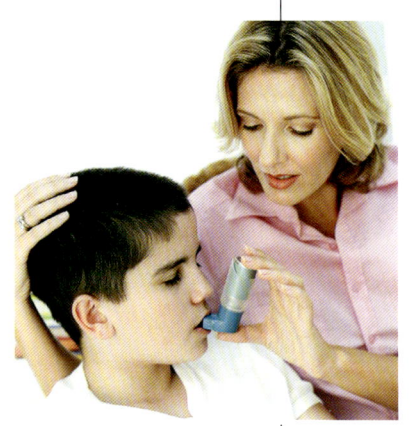

In a recent Australian study, the results were even more encouraging: the children of 616 pregnant women (with a family history of asthma) were randomly selected to observe (or not) a diet enriched in omega-3. These children taking omega-3 (not to excess, because the advice was dietary in nature, without prescription of supplements in capsule form) were significantly less affected by asthma than those of the control group, but without any difference or modification in allergy markers such as patch tests or serum immunoglobulin E levels.

How do the omega-3s act?

The mechanism suggested is as follows: Omega-3s act by substituting themselves for AA in the chain of synthesis of leucotrienes (inflammatory compounds contributing to bronchial spasm). This means that omega-3s would not prevent allergic reaction but would reduce the intensity of the bronchial response to allergens. In other words, omega-3s would not affect the sensitization of subjects (the blood tests testing specific sensitivity to allergens remain positive), but the bronchial tubes would be less reactive (spastic).

Our advice

Clearly, as in the case of joint diseases, we need to generate more information from trials conducted in the early stages of asthmatic disease.

Meanwhile, due to all the other benefits resulting from the rebalancing of our dietary habits, we recommend to all asthmatics at the very least to follow the recommendations drawn up for the prevention of cardiovascular diseases, because one thing is certain: no negative effect on asthma has been observed in any of the trials conducted with severely affected patients.

Chronic bronchitis, and emphysema too!

Other chronic bronchial and inflammatory diseases (notably those resulting from smoking which are often associated with the risk of heart attack) are improved through omega-3 intake, which is another argument in favor of a strategy to increase omega-3s (and reduce omega-6s) in all bronchial pathologies having a spastic ingredient.

And against bronchial spasm in the athlete?

Especially where training is intense, some sports can induce a very troublesome form of bronchospasm. Researchers have tested the hypothesis that omega-3 supplements (about 5 g per day of EPA+DHA) could reduce such bronchospasm. They were right. In this randomized trial, the omega-3s improved pulmonary functions and led to a reduction in the use of bronchodilator medicines.

Protecting oneself against Alzheimer's disease

Senile dementias, especially the terrible Alzheimer's disease, are often considered as cerebral inflammatory diseases. Certain oxidized derivatives of omega-6 and omega-3 fatty acids could be involved in some of these dementias.

Mediterranean diet for the whole world!

For old people, moderate consumption of alcohol - typically of wine (very rich in antioxidants) - is equally recommended to protect the intellectual function while ageing. Inflammatory and degenerative cerebral pathologies therefore appear to be responsive to several types of nutrients, notably alcohol and antioxidants, in addition to omega-3s. It is quite possible that combined approaches with suitable doses could prove more effective than the compartmentalization characteristic of the pharmacological approach - and especially when used for prevention rather than cure.

Again, the same applies to cardiovascular diseases. We must return, therefore, to the Mediterranean diet!

DHA, the target of free radicals

With the ageing of western populations, the number of patients with cerebral degenerative pathologies such as Alzheimer's disease tends to increase exponentially. Although the exact causes of the disease remain unknown, deposits of pro-inflammatory substances have been located in those regions of the brain most damaged by the disease and it seems that anti-inflammatory medicines can delay the onset of symptoms in subjects at risk, or improve some symptoms for patients already affected by the disease.

According to some researchers, the oxidized derivatives of AA (omega-6) and of DHA (omega-3) are implicated in some dementias (AA and DHA are the principal fatty acids of the brain). The oxidized derivatives of DHA, in particular, have been discovered in large quantities in the brains of Alzheimer's patients, in contrast to subjects of the same age unaffected by this disease. For now it is impossible to say whether these products of the oxidative degradation of DHA are the cause or the effect of Alzheimer's disease, or to determine the relation that exists with symptoms of cognitive deficiency.

Protecting DHA

These data suggest that cerebral DHA is the target of oxidative attack and that Alzheimer's patients are unable to protect their DHA. This loss of DHA, whether primary (cause of the disease) or secondary (a consequence of the disease) can only contribute to the aggravation of the symptoms, which are reminiscent of accelerated ageing.

Studies have shown, moreover, that certain antioxidant vitamins (especially vitamin E) could delay or prevent the onset of Alzheimer's disease. We await confirmation of these studies.

While we await new research, a prudent approach to reducing the risk of dementia is to increase one's intake of omega-3 fatty acids.

Because it is clearly important to defend our cerebral DHA against oxidative attack, it would also be wise to:
- reduce intake of omega-6 fatty acids which are the first targets of lipid oxidation and active propagators of radical species and oxidative stress,
- to increase one's intake of oleic acid (powerful lipid antioxidant),
- to increase one's intake of natural antioxidants and of vitamin B, especially folic acid.

Alzheimer's: dramatic symptoms

These dementias are characterized by a more or less rapid - but inescapable - deterioration of cognitive capacity. Memory disorders are the most dramatic and sometimes the most tragic symptoms, and these patients become progressively more dependent on those around them.

The brain, no longer what it was

Independently of any obvious cerebral inflammatory disease, a person's intellectual functions necessarily deteriorate with age. At least two studies, in France and in the Netherlands, have suggested that omega-6 fatty acids tend to promote this intellectual deterioration (the result of a "normal" ageing process), while omega-3 fatty acids slow it down.

When the colon is the seat of the inflammation

Crohn's disease and hemorrhagic rectocolitis are two very disabling diseases of the digestive tract, often affecting young persons, and sometimes necessitating serious medicinal treatments (corticosteroids) having serious side effects.

Very disabling diseases

Like many inflammatory diseases, Crohn's disease and hemorrhagic rectocolitis manifest themselves in the form of acute attacks interrupted by remissions which may be of long or short duration or total remission. The following are the symptoms: abdominal pains, diarrhea, hemorrhages, fatigue, fever, malnutrition, loss of weight. They can require repeated surgical interventions.

Treatment is aimed, on the one hand, essentially at shortening and relieving the attacks and on the other hand (during remission) at preventing the onset of new attacks. Once the disease has taken hold, the effectiveness of a treatment must be evaluated in accordance with these clinical factors, knowing that the correct solution might simply be to reduce the quantity of anti-inflammatory medicines used during a given period. Other criteria, such as the absence of weight loss, the nutritional condition of patients or other biological parameters, will also help decide the effectiveness or usefulness of a new treatment.

Nothing should be left to chance

There is no standard miracle treatment for these digestive ailments. However, any complementary treatment capable of reducing the frequency, duration and severity of recurrences, as well as reducing the intake of medicines, is obviously of real significance for patients. That said, all the studies published to date have been carried out under an ideology which is typically pharmacological and not nutritional in nature. Nothing is known about the dietary habits of those who took part in the trials and, for example, it is not known whether the patients who did best with omega-3 supplementation were deficient in omega-3 (or overloaded by omega-6).

At least three grams per day!

Although unanimity among doctors and researchers is still lacking, one can say that omega-3 fatty acids have had a positive effect on a number of efficacy parameters, at the doses utilized (about 3 g per day) and when used appropriately (for prevention during remissions). Reduction in the doses of corticosteroids appears particularly important during the phases of activity of hemorrhagic rectocolitis.

Despite the lack of any real consensus on this approach, it seems that increased omega-3 intake is a valuable approach complementing the classical treatment of inflammatory colon diseases. At the very least, it should help reduce the dosage and duration for administration of medicines.

Since no significant side effects need be feared, our position is that no subject involved stands to lose anything by trying out this type of treatment, especially where the aim is prevention, or during the dormant phases of the disease. During the active phases, many "gastro-intestinal" factors may impede this dietary approach (for example a reduction in the digestive absorption of lipids). Again, the issue arises of the value of an integrated nutritional approach for patients, and the primary question must be: are recurrences associated with a deficiency in omega-3?

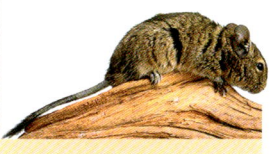

In animals too

Studies conducted on experimental models of inflammatory colitis (using most frequently the rat) confirm the importance of omega-3s in inflammatory colic pathologies. It is true, however, that the experimental models in this area of research do not relate directly to human diseases, which naturally limits the possibilities of extrapolation.

An inflammatory skin disease: psoriasis

This is a very new area of medical research, more or less surrendered to cosmetology specialists. One should therefore be careful to consider only well-founded medical data. Our remarks will be limited to psoriasis, a chronic inflammatory skin disease.

Contrasting results!

Several medical teams have tried to treat patients suffering from psoriasis with omega-3s. Three types of treatment have been tested. Some have used local treatments (ointments or lotions) applied directly onto the lesions, but without success.

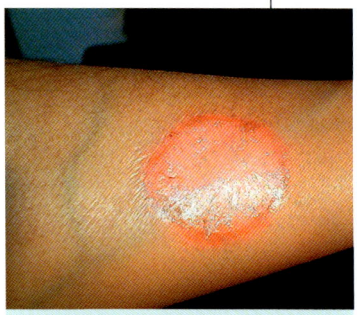

What we know about psoriasis

The very common disease of psoriasis can considerably affect the daily life of patients. They present with scaly lesions and at times very troublesome itching. There are some treatments, notably local (UVB rays, tar treatments, derivatives of vitamin D), but there are common side effects. Apart from a family predisposition (genetic), numerous environmental factors - notably nutritional - appear to play a role during phases of attack or remission of the disease.

Other treatments have used fish oils in the form of capsules, for example, and the results have been inconclusive: some report clear improvements, others clear failure. There are several possible explanations for these inconclusive results: variations in the doses of omega-3, duration of treatment and the clinical condition of patients included in these studies. However, the most plausible explanation is simply that the dietary habits of patients treated in the different trials were basically different. In fact, as we have repeated many times in this book, high consumption of omega-6 fatty acids can inhibit the beneficial effect of omega-3 fatty acids; this is notably the case for metabolic disorders of fatty acids of the skin.

To avoid these methodological problems, German researchers treated their patients with intravenous perfusions of fatty acids. They compared the perfusions of omega-3 fatty acids with perfusions of omega-6 fatty acids. Although only one team has to date published its results, there appears to be no ambiguity: omega-3s rapidly improve the condition of patients with psoriasis, in contrast to omega-6s.

Change now!

While awaiting confirmation of these results, patients suffering from psoriasis have nothing to lose by immediately altering their dietary habits, due to the many other omega-3-related protective effects (especially cardiac) described in this book.

Therefore it is necessary:

1. to consume more fatty fish or even fish oil capsules, because the required doses can be difficult to obtain through ordinary daily consumption of fish,

2. to lower one's intake of omega-6.

The Eskimos again!

As with cardiovascular diseases, inflammatory arthritis or asthma, populations such as the Eskimos, who have a high consumption of omega-3 fatty acids, do not tend to suffer from psoriasis.

Psoriasis and depression

The form of psoriasis occurring in depression treated with lithium deserves mention. Indeed, some depressive syndromes (notably those which respond well to lithium) also seem to improve with omega-3 intake. In these circumstances, omega-3s appear to be winners in three ways: they can help treat depression and also psoriasis following treatment by lithium; moreover, by their effect on depression they can result in a reduction of the dose of lithium, thereby helping to further reduce the cutaneous lesions of psoriasis.

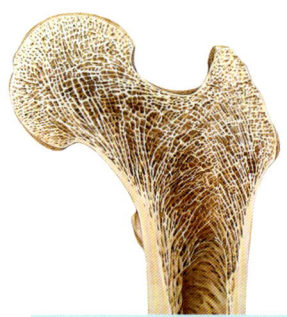

Osteoporosis, an inflammatory bone disease

The life of bones

Our bones are made from a material which continuously renews itself throughout life. The following are very important periods in life for the establishment and maintenance of what may be called our "bone capita": infancy, adolescence, post-menopause for women, old age. Our bone capital depends on a balance between those factors implicated in bone construction (controlled by cells called osteoblasts) and other factors which destroy our bones (the principal cells implicated are known as osteoclasts).

With the ageing of western populations, osteoporosis has become a problem of public health. The formation and growth of bone and the maintenance of a healthy skeleton while ageing depends on many factors, among which are the derivatives of omega-3s.

Bone is a tissue which continuously renews itself (*see box*). This formation-destruction process depends on numerous factors: hormones (estrogen, insulin, growth hormone, thyroid and parathyroid hormones, glucocorticoids), prostaglandins and leucotrienes (derivatives of omega-3 and omega-6 fatty acids), vitamins (D and K) and local growth factors (among which pro-inflammatory cytokines which are of key importance in post-menopause osteoporosis).

Some environmental factors (physical exercise, exposure to sun, nutrition) and genetic factors are also implicated in this process of bone renewal. The main nutritional factors are calcium, magnesium, potassium, vitamin D and animal proteins.

Omega-3 without delay

The rapid bone loss which occurs in the first years of the menopause is considered to be an **inflammatory bone disease** and depends largely on mediators of inflammation (such as prostaglandins and pro-inflammatory cytokines) which activate processes of bone resorption and whose production depends in part on dietary lipids.

If one's dietary habits throughout life (especially during adolescence to build up bone capital) are known to be of crucial importance in the prevention of osteoporosis, experimental and clinical studies clearly indicate that diets supplemented by omega-3 with a low omega-6/omega-3 ratio have a positive effect on the risk of bone loss and osteoporosis.

Omega-3 fatty acids (especially EPA) reduce bone loss by inhibiting the prostaglandins and cytokines generated from arachidonic acid, thereby tilting the balance in favour of bone-formation rather than bone-destruction.

While we await confirmation about the optimal conditions for omega-3 supplementation, women at menopause are recommended not to delay in adopting the dietary habits described in this book which relate to the prevention of cardiovascular diseases. No harmful effect need be feared, and the added potential benefits for the heart, the psyche, the risk of cancer and one's joints (affected by diseases developing especially at the moment of menopause) are so striking that it would be foolish to delay.

Leptin

It is possible that omega-3s interfere with the process of bone formation/destruction by acting on leptin (a hormone produced by the adipose tissue): leptin appears to inhibit bone formation and omega-3s to inhibit the production of leptin.

The reasons for bone loss

Anorexia, slimming diets for the obese or dietary behavior outside the norm (strict vegetarians) can seriously disrupt bone metabolism and lead to very significant bone loss. Age and associated hormonal changes, however, remain the principal causes of bone loss.

When insulin resists

The role of omega-3 fatty acids in diabetes and the so-called "pre-diabetic" syndromes is controversial. However, there is nothing to prevent a diabetic from re-balancing his intake of fatty acids to protect his heart. In fact, it is strongly recommended.

What is insulin resistance?

It is a metabolic disorder where insulin no longer acts efficiently on target cells (in the muscles in particular). It results in poor regulation of blood glucose (diabetes syndromes) or excessive concentrations of insulin, which is generally associated with a myriad of biological disorders (relating to blood lipid imbalance) or physiological disorders (for example overweight or obesity, high blood pressure). According to recent American statistics, **one person in six** in the United States is said to be affected by metabolic syndrome!

Some studies have shown a deterioration of certain biological parameters (fasting glycemia) with high doses of omega-3. In other studies, these modifications were absent or only transitory. There is no clear explanation for these differences, but the existence of a diabetes syndrome or disease is not a counter-indication for the re-balancing of omega-6 and omega-3 intake, especially in the context of cardio-vascular disease prevention. Indeed, diabetics should be considered as coronary patients because the risk of a first heart attack, for a non-coronary diabetic, is more or less the same as the risk of a second heart attack for a diagnosed coronary patient. These observations do not relate solely to insulin-dependent diabetes (juvenile diabetes or again, type I diabetes), but also to type II diabetes (adult-onset) which is much more frequent in rich countries, than in poor countries.

Moreover, it is better to address this question in the context of "metabolic syndrome" (also called "syndrome X") which covers a range of disorders having in common a metabolic peculiarity called "**insulin resistance**" (*read box*).

Resistance to insulin results from chronic inflammation

Recent studies indicate that insulin resistance is in part the **result** (and not the cause) of chronic inflammation. Chronic inflammation is itself dependent on our dietary habits (see page 55). It appears omega-3 fatty acids inhibit the harmful effect of the principal inflammation mediators on insulin resistance.

The epidemiological and experimental data suggest a theory according to which it is preferable to reduce consumption of saturated fats and *trans* fatty acids (those to be found in hydrogenated fats as well as in many industrial foods and in some margarines), to increase monounsaturated fats (canola and olive) and to increase omega-3s to the detriment of omega-6s.

It appears, therefore, that metabolic syndrome responds to the same kind of dietary strategy described in preceding chapters, the fundamental point being to achieve a balance of omega-6/omega-3 intake (increase of omega-3s, reduction of omega-6s).

How much omega-3 for the heart of diabetics?

Epidemiological studies show that to obtain equivalent heart protection, diabetics require a much greater intake of omega-3 than non-diabetics. On average, the best-protected diabetics consumed five portions of fish per week, equivalent to about 2 g per day of EPA+DHA, without counting intake of ALA. This crucially important information is absent from the dietary recommendations given to diabetics.

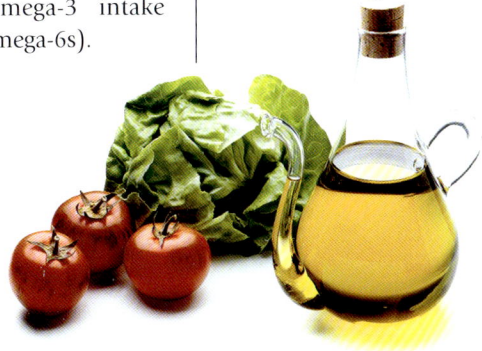

Obesity: From paradox to catastrophe!

Obesity in adults and children has easily become one of the major health problems in western countries, as well as in the comfortable classes of emerging countries, including China and India. This obesity epidemic is an integral part of the global epidemic of metabolic syndrome.

The problem goes back to the cradle

Many experts believe that the source of the current problem is located above all in the way of life (sedentary lifestyle) and the dietary habits of the new generations, going back almost as far as the cradle. Among dietary theories (there are several and they are not mutually exclusive), the most important relates, once again, to the equilibrium between omega-6s and omega-3s. The story begins very early in infancy because several studies have shown a link between the way babies were fed (breast-feeding, formula observing the omega-3/omega-6 balance or otherwise) and differences in weight-gain. In a nutshell: omega-3s have little or no effect on weight-gain, while omega-6s significantly accelerate weight-gain, which is worrying.

More exercise

To overcome overweight, it is essential to increase the level of one's physical activity and to balance the intake of calories (nutrition) with the output or expenditure of calories (exercise) To lose weight, output should be greater than intake.

Is a baby who grows and gains weight quickly really a healthy baby?

The paradox is that these differences in effects on the growth of babies nourished on maternal milk are viewed somewhat negatively by nutritionists, in comparison with omega-3s. We are always delighted to see "our little darlings" grow quickly, all the more so if they are chubby-cheeked; it means, after all, that they are being fed well by good parents! Is this a serious mistake, and is slower growth preferable for our babies (including premature babies)? This question demands an urgent reply, but somebody has to ask it in the first place!

Experimental studies using different animal models which examine the effect of essential fatty acids on growth, are going in the same direction. Omega-6s are believed to favor a general acceleration of growth while omega-3s are neutral in this regard, raising a doubt as to whether they can help babies to grow in a healthy way.

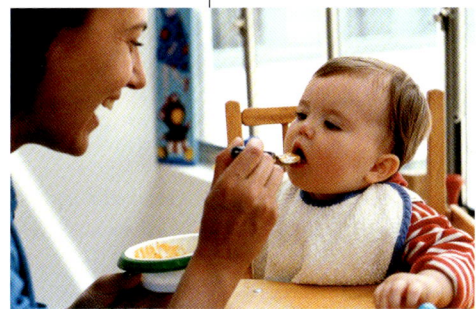

Obesity, a disease programmed from the early months of life

Some scientists strongly defend the theory that too much omega-6 and not enough omega-3, during the key periods of gestation and lactation, favor adipogenesis and the subsequent development of adipose tissue, in other words the differentiation and then the multiplication of specialized cells called adipocytes. These are the cells which accumulate lipids in our organism and are responsible for obesity. For these researchers, the first few months of life (including in the womb) are a critical period during which future obesity may be programmed (or otherwise). The persistence during childhood and into adulthood of a surfeit of omega-6 and a deficit of omega-3 aggravates the problem because in this dietary environment, the adipocytes will only accumulate more lipids.

OMEGA-3s FOR THE BRAIN...
...of the baby

Scientific research on dietary fatty acids during pregnancy and their impact on the health of the fetus is still in its infancy. But this is no reason to delay the implementation of measures necessary to correct deficiencies and imbalances.

Two fatty acids are important for your baby: DHA and AA

A consensus exists today on the importance of DHA for the growth of the fetus (and of the infant) and for the optimal development of the central nervous system. There is more or less general agreement also on the need for arachidonic acid (AA) and a proper balance to exist between DHA and AA. Experimental and clinical studies are fundamental and in a nutshell, we can say that **AA** is essential for **growth** parameters (weight, height, cranial perimeter, *see pages 73-74*) while **DHA** is crucial to the physiology of vision (the retina), to neuronal functions (cognitive) and to the metabolism of chemical messengers in the brain.

DHA, not always in sufficient quantity

The problem is to know what quantities of omega-3 are required during a normal pregnancy and during lactation for a new-born. Paradoxically, there are more data available on the needs of the fetus and the new-born than on the needs of the mother, even

---

For future mothers, canola oil is not enough

Be careful: a vegetable soybean oil or canola oil supplement for the mother (rich in ALA but poor in DHA) will not generate increased DHA concentrations in maternal milk. DHA should therefore be taken either in the form of fatty fish, in the form of eggs from chickens fed on flaxseed (Country Hen) or in the form of dietary supplements rich in DHA.

though it is the mother who nourishes her fetus, and then her baby if she breast-feeds. The fatty acid composition of amniotic fluid and of maternal milk is highly dependent on the fatty acid intake of the mother. Happily, she also has her reserves but it is not certain that they are always enough. These reserves depend on her dietary habits prior to pregnancy – ultimately, in other words, on her family's way of life when she was only a girl.

Omega-3 supplementation for pregnant women is necessary

Some scientists believe that many women should receive supplements during pregnancy to ensure optimal growth and especially normal brain development of the fetus. Should special dietary recommendations be made for pregnant women, possibly including the prescription of dietary supplements?

The response is a double positive: **Yes**, young women should correct the imbalances revealed in the general population and **yes**, as a precaution, they should be prescribed dietary supplements. Very large doses of omega-3 are not necessary (as in inflammatory diseases), but instead the moderate doses recommended for cardiovascular diseases: this helps to avoid disrupting the metabolism of AA which appears to play an important role in growth of the fetus and the new-born. This strategy is a prudent but minimal one.

> **It is crucial that the woman who is or may become pregnant avoids an impoverished diet and in particular obtains nutrients such as folic acid (vitamin B9) and omega-3 fatty acids.**

Omega-3s for the brain...
...of the mother

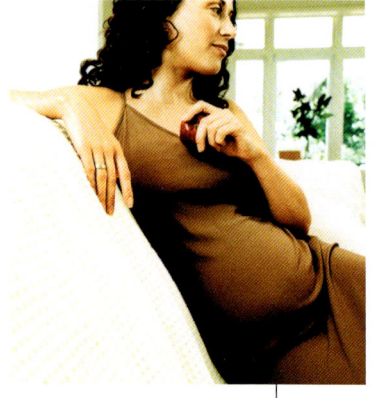

Apart from postnatal depression, a prudent and balanced diet for the pregnant woman should help control a number of pregnancy complications, improve some physiological parameters of the infant and even prevent diseases in the future adult.

More omega-3s, fewer complications

Omega-3 supplementation could prevent the occurrence of certain complications during pregnancy (hypertension, eclampsia) or after pregnancy, especially post-partum maternal depression (and its more attenuated forms sometimes referred to as "baby blues"). This depression could be the consequence of omega-3 depletion in the mother whose reserves (including neurological) would have been used to benefit the developing nervous system of the fetus.

Fewer premature deliveries

Several quality randomized trials have shown that omega-3 supplementation resulted in reduced risk of premature delivery, longer duration of pregnancy (by a few days on average) and increased birth weight. Epidemiological studies carried out on fish consumption confirm this by showing that women consuming low quantities of fish have a distinctly higher risk of premature delivery and low birth weight for their baby.

The concept of transgenerational medicine

The way of life of a generation can have an impact on the health of subsequent generations. That, in a nutshell, is the concept of transgenerational medicine. For any given generation, the risk of developing diseases such as obesity, diabetes, arterial hypertension and the risk of death from heart disease depends at least in part on the way in which previous generations have managed to protect themselves against these diseases. The social and ethical implications of this concept are significant.

In the same way, women consuming average quantities of fish (one portion three times per week) during their pregnancy tend to give birth to infants whose neurological development will be, at least to the 15th month, more sophisticated than that of babies whose mothers never consumed fish. In all likelihood, it is the omega-3s contained in fish which produce these highly beneficial effects.

When fatty acids are put in the baby's bottle

The results of randomized trials testing milk enriched in DHA+AA in infants born at full term have not always been concordant in terms of neurological development, leaving some doubt about the real value of adding such fatty acids to formula. On the other hand, recent studies have shown that the addition of DHA+AA to formula had favorable effects on blood pressure measured at six years of age.

With premature babies, the value of supplementation by fatty acids with 20 to 22 carbon atoms appears to be proven, but it is better to combine AA+DHA. According to the studies published, a supplement using only DHA could delay growth, whereas for premature babies weighing under 1800 g, a combined supplementation of DHA+AA appears to have a definite positive effect on various parameters of neurological development.

> ### Why is the "growth" parameter so important?
>
> Because a considerable number of highly concordant epidemiological studies have shown that there is a relation between birth weight and subsequent development of several chronic diseases, notably obesity, diabetes and arterial hypertension. Therefore, not only is birth weight an indicator of the newborn's state of health and nutrition, but it may also be a long-term prognostic factor. In other words, low birth weight testifies to a certain degree of malnutrition and, paradoxically, increases the subsequent risk of diseases such as diabetes or metabolic syndromes.

The revolution of omega-3s in psychiatry

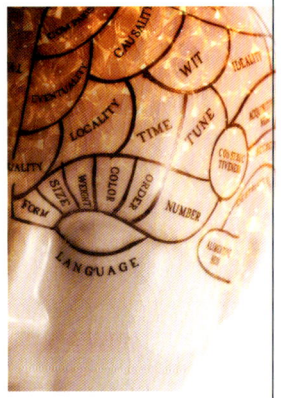

The "rediscovery" of a relationship between mental diseases and omega-3s, after publication of the book *The Instinct To Heal* by David Servan Schreiber, has had the considerable double advantage of revealing the existence of these fatty acids to the general public and making the medical profession realize that our diet can have a genuine impact on our state of psychic health.

Omega-3 and brain: a multitude of data

These days we are bombarded by an incredible number of reports and studies on omega-3s and the brain. They cover practically the whole spectrum of this scientific and medical field, almost as if thousands of laboratories and scientists had been working on these questions for decades, excluding no psychiatric pathologies from their gaze: from suicidal depression to schizophrenia, from personality disorder to the more common emotional and seasonal changes. Well, perhaps that's an exaggeration! In reality, numerous scientists had been researching these questions in the shadows, and the medical and scientific output has in many cases, surprisingly, been substantial and impressive. Having said that, it is now necessary to sort through all this research data to find out how much of it can stand up to scrutiny, and to reject theories and hypotheses which fail to do so. This will be a difficult and time-consuming task, achievable only through the rigorous and honest application of first-rate scientists.

From revelation to discoveries

At a certain point, scientists became suddenly aware that our brain was extremely rich in omega-3 and that its normal development during the fetal and infancy period - and its optimal functioning from then on – in fact depended at least in part on our intake of omega-3. The other revelations about the importance of these fatty acids for cardiac disease, cancer, asthma and inflammatory diseases

– all somewhat incongruous revelations from the contemporary medico-pharmacological point of view - partially concealed the other major discovery: we are generally very deficient in omega-3.

For some fragile or "at risk" groups, one can talk without exaggeration of a genuine physiological scarcity. Unfortunately for this discovery, however, the anticipated media hype has not yet occurred.

A link from cause to effect

The conjunction of this omega-3 deficiency and real epidemic outbreaks of certain psychiatric diseases has led some investigators, especially in the United States, to talk in terms of a possible causal relation. The relative or absolute lack of omega-3 in our neurons (whether continuously or only during the fetal period) might be implicated in the development of certain mental illnesses in both adult and child.

Two aspects of this apparently recent scientific and medical issue must be distinguished.

1. psychiatric illnesses. Clinical investigation is needed, requiring epidemiological data and clinical trials. We will focus here on depression, a true illness of civilization in the view of many experts, and above all a risk factor for suicide;

2. the more basic aspect of cerebral and neuronal development and functioning. We will deal with this second issue only briefly.

Lets sort it out!

These days one finds researchers (especially in the United States) who have very recently become converts to this leading theme, who plunge into new investigations using methods and concepts which prove to be inadequate, but this does not prevent them from publishing their results – sometimes with much fanfare – only to sow more confusion in the area. Not to mention a whole class of new experts (and lecturers) who appear before the media in a highly learned manner, to express their opinions and impressions on the subject...

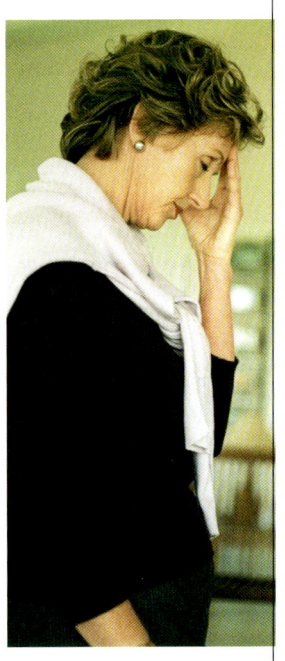

An illness of society: depression

Currently, depression is the most researched illness in psychiatry from the point of view of the potential benefits of omega-3 fatty acids. In the US, an estimated 5.3% of adults or 17 million people suffer from depression; In Europe, roughly 10 to 20 % of Europeans are affected by depressive syndromes and France is one of the most affected countries.

A veritable epidemic

One of the tragic but as yet underestimated aspects of this "epidemic" is that these syndromes are affecting younger and younger subjects and that depression in children is no longer rare. Depression has a catastrophic impact in terms of occupational disability and social cost.

The epidemic of depression in the west didn't just fall out of the sky, it was the necessary consequence of the recent change in our environment and our way of life. Certainly, there are family predispositions (genetic) to depression - as with cardiovascular diseases - but these hardly explain this upsurge in the epidemic.

Recent changes in our dietary habits have certainly contributed to this unexpected depression epidemic.

Omega-3/omega-6 imbalance implicated

It is certainly not the only causal factor involved, for all chronic human diseases are multi-factorial.

Nevertheless, the deficiency in omega-3 and excess of omega-6 in our current diets can only add fuel to the epidemic. This probably occurs in a way that varies from one patient to the other and one country to the other.

Aside from the genetic factor in depression (some families are predisposed to depression), the other factors which relate to lifestyle are often associated with diet and amount to one and the same factor; for instance, work stress is a factor in depression often linked with deplorable eating habits. Occupational stress, which often goes hand-in-hand with family stress, is significant in western countries where daily life in the firm, the office, the factory and the workshop is too often characterized by conflict and stress.

Objective: to cure

Depression is not one single illness, even if very different illnesses are generally categorized under the one label. In the past, depression was classified in terms of the circumstances in which it arose and in terms of the risk of suicide. If it occurred in reaction to a life trauma, one spoke of reactive depression. If it occurred without any apparent cause, one spoke of endogenous depression. Today, even if these old concepts have not been completely abandoned, the main priority appears to be to determine which of a variety of different medicines will help a particular patient. This is the exclusively pharmacological vision of psychiatry.

Too often, the doctor takes on the role of a prescriber of medicines which he has at his disposal, medicines with definite side effects which often lead to dependency. We disagree strongly with the psychoanalytic vision which claims to treat an illness by setting up a specific relation between the patient and the therapist - a form of therapy which is often long and costly. The dream of all people affected by one of these illnesses is obviously to find healing and therefore in consequence, as David Servan-Schreiber writes, to "get rid of" these two very forms of dependency: medicine and the psychoanalyst. The book proved to be very successful!

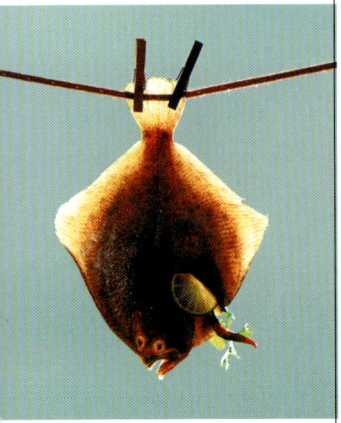

Counter depression by eating fish

Modern psychiatry is replete with shortcomings. But it has finally, especially in the United States, entered the era of modern medicine with its biological and epidemiological approaches.

What epidemiology tells us

The first harvest of information is not very significant, but it seems very clear that populations having a high to moderate consumption of fish are at lower risk of severe depression than those who consume little or no fish. Similar tendencies have been described in relation to alpha-linolenic acid (ALA). Ignoring these tendencies will do nothing to improve the prevalence of depression.

Finally, we now know that depressed people have low concentrations of omega-3 in their blood and in their cells, in contrast to people who do not suffer from depression.

Like heart diseases

The biological profiles of depressed people are similar, therefore, to those observed in patients suffering from cardiovascular diseases. This point is crucial because there is a strong correlation between the risk of heart attack and the risk of depression. This cannot be down to chance. For a long time, it was believed that this association of patholo-

Depression and cardiopathies: danger!

Both pathologies together generate a very high risk of dying from a bad heart! To repeat, therefore: it is a matter of utmost urgency to correct deficiencies in omega-3 (and excesses of omega-6) which are clearly associated with both pathologies and which mutually reinforce one another.

Correcting omega-3 deficiency is imperative for subjects with depressive syndrome, coronary disease and old age.

gies was easy to explain: it was quite natural to be depressed when you were diagnosed with coronary disease, with all the associated risks of sudden death that entailed. However, the more likely explanation is that both diseases have common roots: nutrition.

Randomized clinical trials

At least five randomized clinical studies on omega-3s (essentially EPA) have demonstrated beneficial effects for patients with depression.

The researchers were not always operating in the best possible conditions to test out their theory. In fact in some trials, those recruited were very difficult subjects who were resistant to normal medical treatments. The situation was similar in the case of inflammatory diseases and asthma (*see pages 76-80*). The effects of omega-3s are more likely to be beneficial when they are applied to prevention or to patients who are less affected, or when they are applied at the beginning of the disease because, as we have said, omega-3s are not strictly medicines.

Finally, there is always room to debate the methodological aspects of these trials and to maintain exacting scientific standards, but one cannot ignore these data and behave as if they did not exist!

Always remember to reduce omega-6s

We must insist on one issue which has, to date, been totally neglected by neuro-psychiatrists (because they still naively believe that omega-3s are medicines): correction of a deficiency in omega-3 must be linked with a drastic reduction in the intake of omega-6 Linoleic Acid and Arachidonic Acid. For some subjects, even the doubling or tripling of their intake of omega-3 is not significant when set against the very large quantities of omega-6 which they consume on the advice of their doctor, especially to reduce their cholesterol.

It is important to mention, however, that there is one omega-6 fatty acid which has beneficial effects in certain conditions. This fatty acid is Gamma-Linolenic Acid (GLA), and research shows GLA can reduce pain and inflammation associated with rheumatoid arthritis, relieve symptoms of eczema, prevent and in some cases reverse diabetic neuropathy, and play a positive role in some types of cancer. GLA is not a fatty acid commonly found in foods, but it is found in certain plant oils, namely Evening Primrose, Borage, Black Currant and Hemp oil.

The other psychiatric illnesses

Schizophrenia and some behavioral disorders have also been the subject of intensive research relating to omega-3 fatty acids.

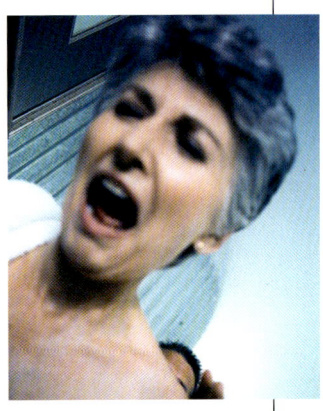

Frequency of personality disorders

According to recent statistics in the United States, it is estimated that about 31 million American adults (15 % of the population) satisfy the typical criteria for these personality disorders. It should be noted that all these millions of people, short of outright mental illness, suffer from significant emotional disabilities and serious social and occupational problems. Paranoia-type syndromes are more common among women while antisocial behavior is more common in men.

Schizophrenia

This devastating mental illness generally occurs at the beginning of adult life. Today, the results are available for five randomized clinical trials where omega-3s were used with schizophrenic patients. Four have produced results which for some symptoms are, to say the least, encouraging. The studies also show that these patients often present a metabolic syndrome (with overweight or obesity and insulin resistance). This suggests that an integrated nutritional approach is necessary and that metabolic and psychiatric disorders may have common roots.

Other relatively more benign syndromes such as personality disorders which are characterized by poorly-controlled aggression and impulsivity as well as signs of depression, have given rise to randomized clinical trials using omega-3s. The results are quite favorable for some syndromes although they require confirmation, while for other more complex syndromes (such as obsessive compulsive disorder), the trials have not had a successful outcome.

Hostile and violent behavior

Several studies carried out in various situations, including prisons, suggest that violence, aggression and hostility especially in young and sometimes drug-addicted persons (cocaine addicts), can be produced by dietary imbalances, especially the total absence of fish (and therefore DHA) from one's diet. A randomized trial in Japan using 1.8 g of DHA in students seems to confirm this sedative (or mood regulating) effect of omega-3s.

Hyperactive child syndrome

In just a few years, this syndrome has become the most frequent of childhood behavioral disorders. It is often associated with symptoms of depression, behavioral disorders and learning disorders (dyslexia and dyspraxia). When it comes to treatment, however, we are still far from a prevention scenario. However, randomized studies suggest that omega-3 supplementation has a role to play.

Auspicious results

Even if we clearly lack a full understanding of the role of omega-3s (and omega-6s) in cognitive function, it is almost certainly significant and in the near future we should be able to alleviate some of the most common psychiatric syndromes - if not to totally abolish them - by applying basic dietary measures.

DHA and EPA do not have the same effects on our neurons

Contrary to the depressive syndromes which appear to be more influenced by EPA than by DHA, personality disorders marked by hostile, impulsive and aggressive behaviors appear to depend more on DHA. That could mean that, in terms of the neuronal functions implicated in behavioral and emotional disorders, not all omega-3 fatty acids have the same effects. Clearly, this is a fundamental theme for researchers which will, no doubt, be promptly elaborated.

Omega-3s for better sight

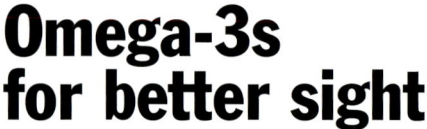

Very long-chain omega-3 fatty acids (DHA and EPA), like arachidonic acid (AA), are the basic compounds of cell membranes of the central nervous system, including cells of the retina.

The retina is rich in omega-3

The cells of the retina are comparable to nervous tissue of the central nervous system. Like neurons, they are very rich in omega-3 fatty acids, especially in DHA.

In several experimental models, when an omega-3 deficiency is induced, visual impairment is systematic and generally not reversible after the diet returns to normal.

Several studies conducted with babies born at full term or premature babies suggest that the parameters of vision are better where DHA is consumed in sufficient and not low quantities. Long-term studies are still necessary, however, to confirm these data.

The immediate ancillary question is whether the omega-3 deficiencies currently observed in our populations have anything in common with some very widespread eye diseases and especially with the well-known age-related macular degeneration (AMD).

AMD: primary cause of poor vision

This disease is due to an alteration in the central area of the retina (the macula) which

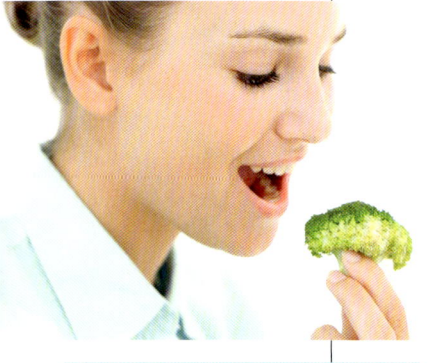

The advice of specialists

Taking into account the totality of biological, epidemiological and clinical data, ophthalmology experts concede that a prudent diet would be rich in vitamins C and E and in carotenoids, especially in xanthrophylls (a lot of spinach, broccoli and eggs) to reduce the risk of AMD. Risk of cataracts can also be reduced because the crystalline lens of the eye is also very sensitive to UV and to oxidative stress. For our part, we recommend DHA supplements very early on, which should be associated with a moderate intake of vitamin E and of selenium.

is responsible for our ability to see detail and color precisely, and thus to read, write and focus on objects. This disease affects millions of people in the United States. Aside from age, there are at least two risk factors for AMD which can be eliminated: smoking and unprotected exposure to the sun. Since both these factors are a major source of oxygen free radicals, and therefore of oxidative stress, an **oxidative theory** of AMD has been advanced.

To date, this theory has withstood its critics because several randomized trials have shown that antioxidant supplements (vitamins, minerals, carotenoids) were capable of delaying the development of AMD.

Is DHA deficiency a cause of AMD?

Because DHA is the principal omega-3 in the retina, it would be interesting to find out if the retinas of patients with AMD contain low levels of DHA. For now, this question has not been answered but there is another disease of the retina, pigmentary retinitis linked with chromosome X (a degenerative disease of the retina similar to AMD), which is associated with serious dysfunction in the metabolism of omega-3s, with a marked deficiency in DHA.

Omega-3s: protective fatty acids

The epidemiological data are fairly clear: consumption of omega-3 fatty acids in fish has a protective effect against AMD. Some studies suggest that saturated fats of animal origin, however, increase the risk. This brings us back to the area of cardiovascular diseases, and if a link can be established with the oxidative theory of AMD mentioned above, one will be bound to conclude that an integrated dietary approach (the Mediterranean-style diet rich in antioxidants and in omega-3s) would be the best way of countering the AMD epidemic.

Randomized trials have yet to establish whether the risk of AMD will decrease when omega-3 deficiencies are corrected. These are currently underway, and we await the results with great interest.

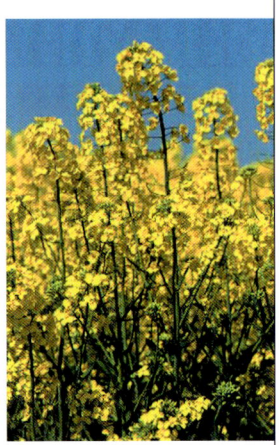

OMEGA-3 PROGRAM

More omega-3 of vegetable origin

To correct your deficiencies in omega-3 you should first of all increase your intake of omega-3 fatty acids of vegetable origin – alpha-linolenic acid or ALA. For this, your table oil is key. Here is some advice for choosing your oil.

Yes, you may heat up your canola oil!

Canola oil may be used cold to prepare vinaigrettes, mayonnaises or to dress a warm dish. It may also be heated up (contrary to what you might read on the label) provided the usual rules are observed: do not smoke the oil, do not exceed a temperature of 350°F for frying, change the frying bath frequently.

ALA exists in vegetable oils such as canola, nuts, soy and other less runny oils such as flaxseed, wheat germ, hemp and mustard. Because one should take into account all the fatty acids present in a particular oil, we strongly recommend canola oil which has the advantage of being rich in monounsaturates (such as olive oil which is, moreover, poor in omega-3) but is relatively poor in saturated fatty acids or omega-6 fatty acids. One tablespoonful of canola oil gives about 1 to 1.5 g of ALA.

- **Canola oil** is easily located in supermarkets and in health food stores. Due to its omega-3 content, it is relatively delicate. Once the bottle is opened, it should be consumed fairly quickly and kept in the shade.

- **Walnut and soybean oils:** although they contain considerable quantities of ALA (about 11 g of ALA per 100 g and 7 g per 100 g for walnut and soybean oils respectively), they have the big

OMEGA-3 PROGRAM

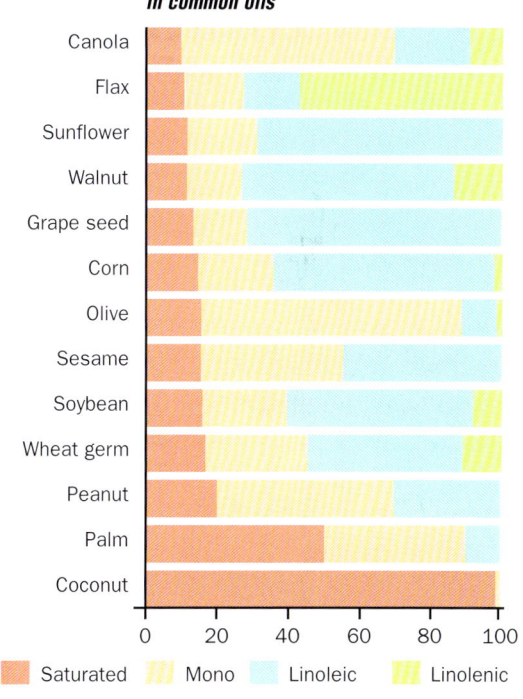

Composition of fatty acids in common oils

disadvantage of being **too rich in omega-6.** For this reason we do not recommend soybean oil. Although walnut oil has undeniable gastronomic qualities, it should only be consumed **occasionally** to accompany a dish.

- **Flaxseed oil** is particularly rich in ALA, with about 53 g per 100 g and it is therefore very delicate, requiring certain precautions to be applied.

- **Olive oil,** symbol of the protective Mediterranean diet, contains low levels of omega-3 fatty acids but is very rich in antioxidants. Besides, it has the huge advantage of being rich in monounsaturated fatty acids (notably oleic acid), poor in saturated fatty acids and also very poor in omega-6. Therefore it the perfect complement of canola oil. By hindering the metabolism of omega-6, it indirectly promotes omega-3.

For all these reasons, we recommend exclusive use of canola and olive oil as the main oils for flavorings and for cooking.

Other sources of ALA

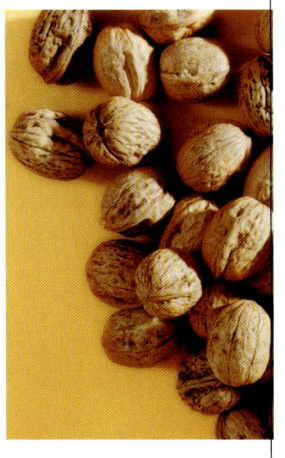

Besides canola oil, other foods should appear more often on the menu: nuts in general and flaxseed.

Nuts

Nuts (fruit with shell) are an important source of oleic acid and, with the exception of coconut, contain low levels of saturated fatty acids. Nuts also contain other nutrients important for human health such as arginine, fiber, minerals (magnesium, potassium or selenium from the Brazil nut), as well as some vitamins such as folic acid (from the Californian walnut) and vitamin E from the hazelnut. For these reasons, all nuts (hazelnuts, almonds, walnuts, pistachio nuts, cashew nuts etc) are recommended. However, **only the classic walnut** (such as the Californian variety) has the advantage of containing significant levels of ALA, 7 g/100 g, so that six or seven walnuts provide about 2 g of ALA, or the minimum quantity of ALA recommended in one day.

The advantage of fruit in comparison with oil is that the fatty acids are, in principle, less adulterated because they come in a natural protective envelope; also fruit contains nutrients other than lipids.

Nuts may be consumed on their own, with bread, cheese, included in cake recipes, breads, unsweetened cakes, added to salads or prepared in walnut pestos, where the classic pine nuts are substituted with walnuts.

What is our daily requirement for ALA?

An average of two grams is generally considered sufficient for an adult weighing 150 pounds. A heavier or more physically active person will naturally require a higher intake. 3 to 4 g per day is a moderate intake that covers your needs and ensures optimal health. Increase this quantity if you do not consume fatty fish or if you do not take omega-3 fatty acid supplements of marine origin (EPA + DHA), because ALA will be the principal source of this family of essential nutrients.

Flaxseed

This is also an excellent source of ALA, with about 3 g of ALA per tablespoon. It can be found in health food stores or in shops selling natural or organic products. You can purchase milled seeds or crush whole seeds on your own and sprinkle on your salads and breakfast cereals or you can add it to flour when making a sweet or unsweetened cake. It is better to keep the milled flaxseeds in the refrigerator and away from sunlight to protect it from oxidation and conserve its goodness. You can also take liquid flax oil or flax oil capsules.

Average content of alpha-linolenic acid (ALA) in certain foods

Foods 1 tablespoonful *	Alpha-Linolenic Acid (ALA)
Canola oil	1 to 1.5 g
Hazelnut oil	1.1 to 1.6 g
Flaxseed oil	5 to 8 g
Ground linseed	1.8 to 2.2 g
Crushed hazelnuts	0.5 to 0.8 g
Enriched egg*	0.4 to 0.6 g per egg
Purslane	0.4 g per 100 g

* The values indicated may vary because the biochemical composition of the foods may vary from one batch to another and one year to another.

Other foods can contribute to one's intake of ALA:

• margarines and other spreads,
• certain green leafy vegetables such as purslane,
• eggs or other products from animals fed on foodstuffs enriched in omega-3 fatty acids,
• Bread made with flour enriched with flaxseed or chia seed.

Animals fed on fresh grass in Spring and Summer on mountain pastures yield milk which is richer in omega-3 fatty acids; cheese made from this milk is to be preferred as it is richer in ALA.

Lastly, some dietary supplements contain ALA.

More omega-3 of marine origin

EPA and DHA are to be found mainly in products of marine origin, especially fatty fish.

Tuna, a fish with a problem

Our lethal civilization produces waste which it then dumps en masse into the sea: this waste is concentrated in the tuna fish which, like other large and long-lived sea fish, are at the end of the marine food chain. In some countries, pregnant women are recommended to avoid consumption of such fish.

Some eggs are a good source of DHA

The eggs of chickens, fed on flaxseed grain or on a natural foodstuff rich in omega-3 fatty acids (Country Hen), can contribute to one's intake of very long-chain omega-3 fatty acids, especially of DHA. Each extra large Country Hen egg contains about 300 mg of DHA.

A minimum of two to three portions of fatty fish per week

Although lipid content varies a lot for the same fish, an intake of two to three portions of fatty fish per week will guarantee an average intake of 1 g of EPA+DHA per day. This is the minimum recommended quantity for cardiac protection. Greater quantities (at least 2 g per day) are not harmful and certainly ensure better protection for people with a high risk of cardiac diseases, such as diabetics. For the latter, the epidemiological data suggests that the best protection is to consume at least five portions of fish per week. Since this could present difficulties from a gastronomic point of view, depending on the country concerned, a more practical way of achieving this result might be to take omega-3 capsules!

Fatty fish are certainly to be found in our supermarkets: salmon, mackerel, tuna, herring, sardine, trout, anchovy, eel. Since omega-3 fatty acids are very sensitive to oxidation, one should be careful to ensure that the fish being sold is fresh.

Smoked, frozen or canned?

These fish may be consumed smoked, frozen or canned. Certainly, the omega-3 fatty acid content may be lower than that of fresh fish (in particular for smoked or frozen fish) but at least they allow you to vary your meals.

There is a wide variety of products in the big supermarkets and specialized shops: smoked salmon and trout, smoked fillets of herring or mackerel, sardines in olive oil, water-packed tuna or tuna in olive oil etc.

Do not forget that fish canned in oil should be exclusively in either canola oil or olive oil. Also, if you are buying water-packed tuna, choose white albacore tuna over chunk light tuna, a low-fat tuna with less omega-3.

Wild or farmed?

Finally, there is no reason not to have fish from properly regulated fish farms. Their omega-3 content is the same as wild fish and they are often fresher at point of sale. Moreover, there is a lower risk of strong concentrations of pesticides, dioxins, and heavy metals in comparison with wild fish because marine farms in general observe strict ecological guidelines.

Lastly, dietary supplements in the form of capsules can be beneficial - if not absolutely essential - to complete one's intake of EPA+DHA.

EPA + DHA content of certain fish products

Fish product	EPA + DHA in g per 100 g of food
Fatty fish	
Anchovy, eel	1.4
Trout	1.6
Scottish smoked salmon	2.1
Atlantic salmon	2.6
Mediterranean red tuna	2.6
Sardine	3.7
Herring	4.1
Mackerel	4.7
Lean fish and shellfish	
Whiting, sole, crayfish	0.1
Cod, monkfish, lobster	0.2
Perch, crab	0.3
Shrimp	0.4
Albacore tuna in water	0.6

NB : the total fat content and fatty acid composition of the fish vary considerably for any given species These depend on the fishing location, the season and the feeding methods used for farmed fish. This explains why values vary considerably from one composition table to another. For example, the total fatty content of sardines may vary between 1.2% in March to 18.4% in September. (High values are given above)

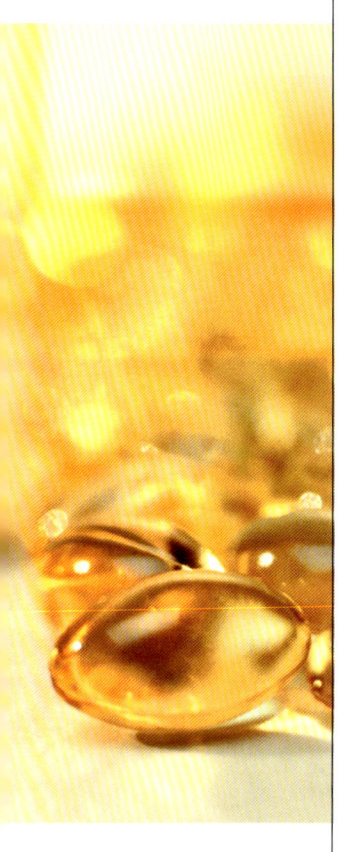

How to enrich one's food intake with omega-3 fatty acids?

If we are to follow the natural model tried and tested in Japan, we would eat fatty fish twice a day. We should take Japan as a model because the Japanese have the lowest rate in the world of cardiovascular diseases, cancer and even depression. But is this feasible in practice? For the majority of us, probably not. Other solutions are therefore required, the ones we have been proposing throughout this book, as well as in our book The Omega-3 Diet (see page 120).

One alternative to the frantic consumption of fish is to use fish oil capsules; one worthwhile solution is supplements containing mixtures of the principal three omega-3s. They should be taken on an intermittent basis, because the treatment should vary in accordance with the dietary habits of the family.
For specifically cardiac prevention, one capsule should be taken (3 to 4 per day) which is highly concentrated in fatty acids and with a high content of DHA.

Whatever kind of capsule is taken, one should double-check the quality of oils used in the capsules and the appropriate quantity of antioxidants added (vitamin E at the very least, but other antioxidants can be added such as selenium).

How do you know if you are deficient in omega-3?

One's weekly intake of fish is a good indicator. Unless you eat fatty fish at least twice a week (or take omega-3 supplements), you are probably deficient in DHA and in EPA.

Indeed, average current consumption in western countries of omega-3s of vegetable origin (ALA) probably represents only about one-third to one-half of recommended intake. Therefore unless you consume canola oil, you are probably seriously deficient in ALA. Moreover, if you consume sunflower oil (or corn or grape seed oil) and you are taking an anti-cholesterol medicine, your physiological deficiency will probably be even more serious.

Biological analyses

To understand the extent of your deficiency in omega-3, you can consult your doctor for analysis of the fatty acids in your blood, or even better of your red blood cells. Unfortunately, the standard values applied by the laboratories are inappropriate because they have been defined by reference to the average values measured in seriously deficient populations (such as ours). Therefore it is difficult to interpret these results without recourse to an expert aware of this difficulty. On the other hand, these values tell us nothing about deficiencies which exist in tissues such as the heart and the brain.

Less omega-6

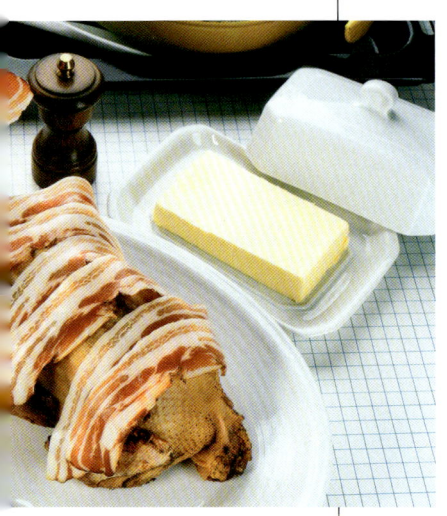

If omega-3s have almost disappeared from our daily food regime, due to the more general availability of industrial foods and the growing scarcity of natural and "wild" products, omega-6s have invaded our refrigerators and cupboards, showing up also in various margarines and oils or in even more insidious forms.

Indeed, because animals are fed on industrial foodstuffs high in omega-6 and low in omega-3, the products that come from them (and not just their fats) - especially dairy products, meats and eggs - have concentrations of omega-6 and omega-3 which simply reflect the way these animals have been fed. Moreover, all industrial foods and pre-packaged dishes generally contain large quantities of omega-6.

How to get rid of them?

The only solution (apart from consumer pressure applied to farmers and manufacturers) is to purchase one's foods in accordance with the following criterion: to systematically reject foods rich in omega-6. And there is no need to worry that your intake of omega-6 will disappear completely because in practice it is very hard to avoid them.

A diet rich in omega-3 but poor in omega-6 has a name: it is the Mediterranean diet which we now briefly describe in the following section (a more complete description of this diet can be found in the book *The Omega-3 Diet*).

Some omega-3 recipes

Walnut bread
(delicious for breakfast!)

Preparation

Mix the egg and then sugar, then all ingredients together.
Pour the mix into a greased cake pan.
Bake for a good hour in the oven at 325° F (check the progress using a knife).

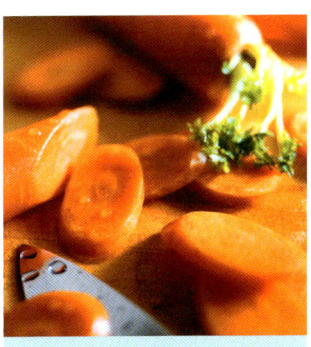

INGREDIENTS

One whole egg
1/2 cup of sugar
1 3/4 cup of flour
1/4 cup of milled flax *
I sachet of yeast
1 pinch of salt
1 cup of chopped walnuts
1 cup of skim or lowfat milk
1 tablespoon of canola oil
(Optional: 2 tablespoons of dried apricots cut into small pieces)

* To prepare milled flax, mill the flaxseeds using a coffee grinder or use FiproFLAX which has been already milled.

INGREDIENTS

2 cups of whole wheat flour
2 cups of powdered sugar
2 teaspoonfuls of yeast
1 level teaspoonful of fine salt
2 teaspoonfuls of powdered cinnamon
3 cups of roughly grated carrots
1 cup of canola oil
4 whole eggs

Carrot cake

Preparation

Preheat oven to 400°F. Oil and lightly flour a cake pan.
Beat the whole eggs with sugar. Add all the other ingredients except the carrots and mix well with a mixer (or by hand).
Added the grated carrots. Mix and pour the preparation into a cake tin and place in the oven.
Bake for about 45 minutes (check the progress using a knife).
You can increase the omega-3 content of this recipe by substituting 3 tablespoonfuls of flour with 3 tablespoonfuls of milled flax (FiproFLAX) or by adding some chopped walnuts.

The Mediterranean diet, a model to follow

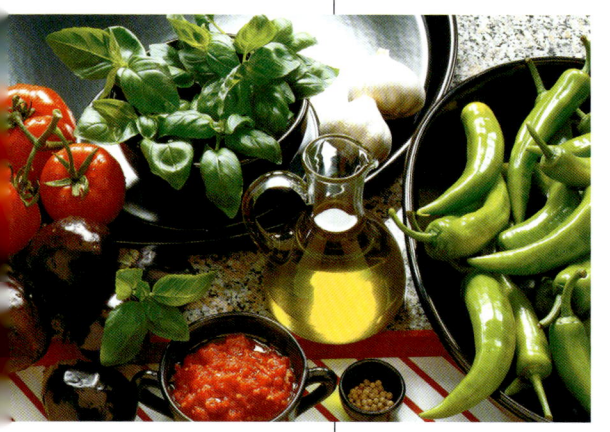

Correcting our deficiency in or lack of omega-3 is imperative if we wish to protect our health. But to get the most out of this correction, other dietary imbalances should be corrected as well.

For cardiovascular protection, in addition to the absolute requirement to reduce one's intake of omega-6, we have stressed the importance of increasing one's intake of monounsaturated fats and reducing one's intake of saturated fats. Moreover, because omega-3s are quite delicate, there should be parallel intake of antioxidants, especially vitamin E and selenium. What is required, therefore, is for our dietary habits to be adapted in an integrated fashion. Clearly, the model to be followed in the West is the Mediterranean diet.

It's healthy and it's good!

Although the word "diet" immediately suggests the idea of restraint or penance, it is nothing of the sort. Traditional Mediterranean dietary customs are staunchly defended by many chefs, as representing the authentic gastronomy of peoples who appreciate the real pleasures of life. From the west of the Mediterranean basin (Spain and Portugal) to the

OMEGA-3 PROGRAM

south (Morocco, Algeria, Tunisia) as far as the east (Middle Eastern cuisine), there is an extraordinary variety of dishes and culinary customs offering genuine pleasure to everyone.

The Mediterranean diet is certainly not the perfect solution for each of us in all parts of the world. The Japanese, for instance, obviously require no outside inspiration! But based on what we know to date, the Mediterranean diet clearly represents the best compromise for good dietary health, without the need to disrupt one's way of life or to travel far and wide in search of solutions, traditional or esoteric.

The Mediterranean diet in broad strokes

It is obviously not possible to set out in a matter of sentences all the characteristics of the traditional Mediterranean diet, as described in our book *The Omega-3 Diet*; all the more so since many aspects of this diet must vary from one region or social class to another.

Still, we can give some general guidelines here, describing the foods themselves rather than the nutrients they contain.

The Mediterraneans eat:

- Many fruits and vegetables in season

- Many dried fruits and vegetables (beans, chickpeas, broad beans depending on region and, on the other hand, raisins and dried apricots, dates, walnuts, almonds, hazelnuts depending on region and season)

- An abundance of garlic, onions, aromatic herbs (basil) and lemon juice used in many recipes

- Many unrefined cereals, above all wheat but also rice

- Almost exclusively olive oil

- Few dairy products, and then only in fermented form (with yogurt and cheese) and from ewe's and goat's milk

- Moderate consumption of animal products, especially eggs, chicken and duck (rabbit in some zones) but not much pork or beef

- Moderate or even high consumption of fish, according to region and season

- Moderate consumption of alcoholic drinks, especially wine while eating and aniseed aperitifs

CONCLUSION

Since Antiquity, men have confused nutrition and health. Only in the modern period, with the development of the pharmaceutical industry and synthetic drugs, has it become possible to separate these two aspects of our daily life.

Without going so far as to reject the benefits of the new and powerful drugs, which have the ability to cure even mortal illnesses (antibiotics, for instance), their use for chronic prevention is an aberration. Such use is in general guided more by the concerns of commerce and marketing than by what is in people's real interest. These practices, in part, are contributing to the escalating health-care costs in this country.

What we should understand is that our health is our own responsibility and no form of medicine (to lower cholesterol or blood pressure) can compensate for the injurious effects of a harmful way of living: smoking, lack of physical exercise or eating habits which contradict the innermost tendencies of physiological and genetic being.

> ## For further information
> We encourage our readers to refer to the following book for practical, dietary applications of the omega-3 fatty acids (or of the Mediterranean diet in general):
>
> **The Omega-3 Diet, the dietary program to save our health**
> By Artémis Simopoulos, Jo Robinson, Dr Michel de Lorgeril and Patricia Salen
> EDP Sciences

A new nutritional medicine is now actually emerging, encouraged by concepts such as the **Mediterranean diet**, or theories like those relating to **omega-3**. In keeping both with the experience of thousands of years and with the latest research, this **new** and scientifically developed medicine is primarily all about prevention. It is also remedial, in that it neutralizes diseases (especially cardiac) which are liable to put life at risk, without appropriate intervention.

GLOSSARY

Adipose tissue: tissue composed of fat cells called adipocytes, situated under the skin or in the abdomen. Adipose tissue represents the largest part of the organism's energy reserve.

Antioxidant: enzymatic substances (often of nutritional origin) and systems which combat oxidation in cells or organic fluids.

Atheroma: deposit of lipids (notably cholesterol) in the lining of an artery.

Arteriosclerosis: hardening and thickening of the arteries following the formation of atheroma plaques or a long period of arterial hypertension (high blood pressure). It can cause a narrowing of the artery capable of obstructing the passage of blood.

Biomarker: biological or biochemical characteristic used to evaluate a physiological condition (for instance, the nutritional health of a person) or pathological condition.

Cachexia: profound state of malnutrition.

Carotid: artery located in the neck carrying blood to the brain.

Coronary: artery supplying blood to the heart muscle.

Cytokine: molecule produced and secreted by various tissues or cells (notably white globules) and involved in the growth and regulation of the immune response system.

Dyslexia: learning difficulties associated with reading and spelling, unrelated to sensory or intellectual deficiency or psychiatric disturbance.

Dyspraxia: psychomotive disorder (sometimes affective), often accompanied by learning difficulties associated with reading, writing and computation.

Implantable defibrillator: device (similar in size to a pacemaker) implanted in the skin which monitors heart rhythm. In cases of malign arrhythmia (serious disorder of the heart rhythm), it is capable of registering the arrhythmia and activating an electric shock (low energy) to correct or eliminate this irregularity of rhythm.

Ion channel: cell membrane space allowing the passage of certain ions (e.g. potassium, calcium). These ion movements produce variations in electric potential in transmembrane ion channels which play a crucial role in the regulation of heart rhythm and contraction and in communication between cells.

Malign ventricular arrhythmia: disorder of the heart rhythm involving problems of cardiac contraction (and the heart pump function), which can be fatal.

Malnourishment: pathological state where the organism's needs for energy or varied nutrients are not being met.

Leucocytes: blood cells also called white globules, different varieties of which play a role in defending the organism against invasive agents.

Leucotriene: substances derived from unsaturated fatty acids which are mediators of inflammation. Leucotrienes are also involved in the regulation of bronchial functions.

Metabolic syndrome or syndrome X: metabolic disorder diagnosed when a person presents at least three of the following symptoms: abdominal obesity, high triglyceride level, excessively low cholesterol-HDL (good cholesterol), hypertension, elevated fasting insulin levels.

Mitochondria: cell organelles whose essential role is to ensure respiration and energy production by cells: It is the cell's lung.

Oxidative stress: condition of molecules and cells subject to the action of free radicals. The level of oxidative stress depends on equilibrium between the quantity of free radicals and the quality of the organism's antioxidant defenses. It can be determined by a certain number of biochemical tests.

Prostaglandins: substances derived from unsaturated fatty acids, having a common biochemical structure of the cyclical type. They are produced naturally by the organism and act as mediator in many physiological and pathological (notably inflammatory) phenomena.

Sudden cardiac death: cardio-respiratory arrest produced generally by a malign ventricular arrhythmia of the ventricular tachycardia or ventricular fibrillation variety. This type of complication may occur at any time during a benign (angina pectoris) or malign (infarction) cardiac crisis.

Trans fatty acid: the term "trans" refers to a particular arrangement within the fatty acid molecule, in contrast with the term "cis", an arrangement which generally applies to fatty acids in their natural state. Trans fatty acids can result from the industrial hydrogenation of vegetable oils and in this case, they are considered harmful to human health.

Thromboxanes: substances derived from unsaturated fatty acids producing the aggregation of blood platelets, the contraction of artery walls and increase in blood pressure.

Ventricular fibrillation: serious abnormal heart rhythm characterized by the disappearance of all coordinated contraction of the ventricles and the appearance of irregular contractions.

BIBLIOGRAPHY

Part 1: the world of omega-3s

Sinclair A. *What is the role of alpha-linolenic acid for mammals?* Lipids 2002;37:1113-23.

Connor WE. *Alpha-linolenic acid in health and disease.* Am J Clin Nutr 1999;69:827-8.

Emken EA. *Metabolism of deuterium-labeled linolenic, linoleic, oleic, stearic and palmitic acid in human subjects.* In Baillie TA, Jones JR Eds. Synthesis and applications of isotopically labeled compounds. Amsterdam: Elsevier Science 1989;713-6.

Krauss RM. *AHA dietary guidelines: revision 2000.* Circulation 2000;102:2284-99.

Lands WE. *Quantitative effects of dietary polyunsaturated fats on the composition of fatty acids in rat tissues.* Lipids 1990;25:505-16.

Mantzioris E. *Dietary substitution with alpha-linolenic acid-rich vegetable oil increases eicosapentaenoic acid concentration in tissues.* Am J Clin Nutr 1994;59:1304-9.

Serhan CN. *Novel functional sets of lipid-derived mediators with anti-inflammatory actions generated from omega-3 fatty acids via cyclooxygenase 2-non-steroidal anti-inflammatory drugs and transcellular processing.* J Exp Med 2000;192:1197-204.

Part 2: omega-3 and diseases of civilization

Bang H. T*he composition of the Eskimo food in northwestern Greenland.* Am J Clin Nutr 1980;33:2657-61.

Marckmann P. *Fish consumption and coronary heart disease mortality. A systematic review of prospective cohort studies.* Eur J Clin Nutr 1999;53:585-90.

Kromhout D. *Fish consumption and sudden cardiac death.* JAMA 1998;279:65-6.

Sandker GN. *Serum cholesteryl ester fatty acids and their relation with serum lipids in elderly men in Crete and Netherlands.* Eur J Clin Nutr 1993;47:201-8.

Singhal A. *Early origins of cardiovascular disease: is there a unifying hypothesis?* Lancet 2004; 363:1642-45.

Hattersley AT. *The fetal insulin hypothesis: an alternative explanation of the association of low birthweight with diabetes and vascular disease.* Lancet 1999;353:1789-92.

Rudin DO. *The dominant diseases of modernized societies as omega-3 essential fatty acid deficiency syndrome: substrate beriberi.* Med Hypotheses 1982 8:17-47.

Crawford MA. *Fatty-acid ratios in free-living and domestic animals. Possible implications for Atheroma.* Lancet 1968;1:1329-33.

Cordain L. F*atty acid analysis of wild ruminant tissues :evolutionary implications for reducing diet-related chronic disease.* Eur J Clin Nutr 2002;56:181-91.

Part 3: omega-3 and cardiovascular diseases

Leaf A. *Clinical prevention of sudden cardiac death by n-3 polyunsaturated fatty acids and mechanism of prevention of arrhythmias by n-3 fish oils.* Circulation 2003;107:2646-52.

De Lorgeril M, Salen P. *Fish and n-3 fatty acids for the prevention and treatment of coronary heart disease.* Am J Med 2002;112:316-9.

De Lorgeril M, Salen P, al. *Dietary prevention of sudden cardiac death.* Eur Heart J 2002;23:277-85.

Burr ML. *Effects of changes in fat, fish and fibre intakes on death and myocardial reinfarction.: Diet and Reinfarction Trials (DART).* Lancet 1989, 2 :757-761.

Schrepf R. *Immediate effects of n-3 fatty acid infusion on the induction of sustained ventricular tachycardia.* Lancet 2004;363:1441-2.

GISSI-*Prevenzione Investigators. Dietary supplementation with n-3 polyunsaturated fatty acids and vitamin E after myocardial infarction: results of the GISSI-Prevenzione trial.* Lancet. 1999;354:447-55.

De Lorgeril M. *Mediterranean alpha-linolenic acid-rich diet in secondary prevention of coronary heart disease.* Lancet 1994;343:1454-9.

De Lorgeril M, Salen P. *Mediterranean diet, traditional risk factors and the rate of cardiovascular complications after myocardial infarction. Final report of the Lyon Diet Heart Study.* Circulation 1999;99:779-85.

Kris-Etherton P. *Lyon Diet Heart Study. Benefits of a Mediterranean-style, National Cholesterol Education Program/American Heart Association step I dietary pattern on cardiovascular disease.* Circulation 2001;103:1823-5.

Thies F. *Association of n-3 polyunsaturated fatty acids with stability of atherosclerotic plaques: a randomized controlled study.* Lancet 2003;361:477-85.

McLennan PL. *The cardiovascular protective role of docosahexaenoic acid.* Eur J Pharmacol 1996;300:83-9.

Christensen JH. *Heart rate variability and fatty acid content of blood cell: a dose-response study with n-3 fatty acids.* Am J Clin Nutr. 1999;70:331-7.

Oskarson HJ. *Dietary fish oil supplementation reduces myocardial infarct size in a canine model of ischemia and reperfusion.* J Am Coll Cardiol 1993;21:1280-5.

Daviglus ML. *Fish consumption and the 30-year risk of fatal myocardial infarction.* N Engl J Med 1997;336:1046-53.

Part 4: omega-3 and cancers

Rose DP. *Dietary fatty acids and cancer.* Am J Clin Nutr 1997;66(suppl):998-1003.

Carroll KK. *Experimental evidence of dietary factors and hormone-dependent cancers.* Cancer Res 1975;35:3374-83.

Susanna C. *Dietary long-chain n-3 fatty acids for the prevention of cancer: a review of potential mechanisms.* Am J Clin Nutr 2004;79:935-45.

Bougnoux P. *N-3 polyunsaturated Fatty acids and cancer.* Curr Opin Clin Nutr Metab Care 1999;2:121-6.

Pearce ML. *Incidence of cancer in men on a diet high in polyunsaturated fat.* Lancet 1971;1:464-7.

De Lorgeril M, Salen P. *Mediterranean dietary pattern in a randomized trial. Prolonged survival and possible reduced cancer rate.* Arch Intern Med 1998;158:1181-7.

Freeman VL. *Prostatic levels of fatty acids and the histopathology of localized prostate cancer.* J. Urol. 2000;164:2168-72.

De Lorgeril M, Salen P. α-*Linolenic acid, coronary heart disease and prostate cancer.* J Nutr 2004 (in press).

Part 5: omega-3 and inflammatory diseases

Mori TA. *Docosahexanoic acid, but not eicosapentaenoic acid, lowers ambulatory blood pressure and heart rate in humans.* Hypertension 1999;34:253-60.

Woodman RJ. *Effects of purified eicosapentaenoic and docosahexaenoic acids on glycemic control, blood pressure, and serum lipids in type 2 diabetic patients with treated hypertension.* Am J Clin Nutr 2002;76:1007-15.

Storlien LH. *Polyunsaturated fatty acids, membranc function, and mctabolic diseases such as obesity and diabetes.* Curr Opin Clin Nutr Metab Care 1998;1:559-63.

Pikkujamsa SM. *Heart rate variability and baroreflex sensitivity in hypertensive subjects with and without metabolic features of insulin resistance syndrome.* Am J Hypertens 1998;11:523-31.

Kataoka M. *Low heart rate variability is a risk factor for sudden cardiac death in type 2 diabetics.* Diabetes Res Clin Pract 2004;64:51-8.

Hu FB. *Fish and long-chain n-3 fatty acid intake and risk of coronary heart disease and total mortality in diabetic women.* Circulation 2003;107:1852-7.

Massiera F. *Arachidonic acid and prostacyclin signalling promote adipose tissue development: a human health concern?* J Lipid Res 2003;44:271-9.

Clement K. *Weight loss regulates inflammation-related genes in white adipose tissue of obese subjects.* FASEB J 2004;18:1657-69.

Robinson D. *Suppression of autoimmune disease by dietary n-3 fatty acid.* J Lipid Res. 1993 34:1435-44.

Michael J. *Dietary polyunsaturated fatty acids and inflammatory mediator production.* Am J Clin Nutr 2000;71:343-8.

Schwartz J. *Role of polyunsaturated fatty acids in lung disease.* Am J Clin Nutr 2000;71:393-6.

Cleland L. *Omega-6/Omega-3 fatty acids and arthritis.* World Rev Nutr Diet. 2003;92:152-68.

Morris M. *Consumption of fish and n-3 fatty acids and risk of incident Alzheimer disease.* Arch Neurol. 2003; 60:940-6.

Belluzzi A. *Effect of an enteric-coated fish oil preparation on relapses in Crohn's disease.* N Eng J Med. 1996; 334:1557-60.

Mayser P. *N-3 fatty acids in psoriasis.* Br J Nutr 2002; 87 suppl 1:77-82.

Nagakura T. *Dietary supplementation with fish oil rich in omega-3 polyunsaturated fatty acids in children with bronchial asthma.* Eur Respir J 2000; 16:861-5.

Winnicki M. *Fish-rich diet, leptin, and body mass.* Circulation 2002;106:289-91.

Part 6: omega-3, neurons and brain

Coste TC. *Neuroprotective effect of docosahexaenoic acid-enriched phospholipids in experimental diabetic neuropathy.* Diabetes 2003;52:2578-85.

Connor W. *Essential fatty acids: the importance of n-3 fatty acids in the retina and brain.* Nutr Rev 1992;50:21-9.

Neuringer M. *Biochemical and functional effects of prenatal and postnatal omega-3 fatty acid deficiency on retina and brain in rhesus monkeys.* Proc Natl Acad Sci USA 1986;83:4021-5.

Lauritzen I. *Polyunsaturated acids are potent neuroprotectors.* EMBO J 2000; 19:1784-93.

Frasure-Smith N. *Major depression is associated with lower omega-3 fatty acid levels in patients with recent acute coronary syndromes.* Biol Psychiatry 2004; 55:891-6.

Adams P. *Arachidonic acid to eicosapentaenoic acid ratio in blood correlates positively with clinical symptoms of depression.* Lipids 1996; 31:157-61.

Stoll A. *Omega-3 fatty acids in bipolar disorder. A preliminary double-blind, placebo-contolled trial.* Arch Gen Psychiatry 1999;56:407-12.

Peet M. *A dose-ranging study of the effects of ethyl-eicosapentaenoate in patients with ongoing depression despite apparently adequate treatment with standard drugs.* Arch Gen Psychiatry 2002;59:913-9.

Hibbeln JR. *Fish consumption and major depression.* Lancet 1998;351:1213.

Fenton W. *A placebo-controlled trial of omega-3 fatty acid (ethyl eicosapentaenoic) supplementation for residual symptoms and cognitive impairment in schizophrenia.* Am J Psychiatry 2001;158:2071-4.

Hamazaki T. *The effect of docosahexaenoic acid on aggression in young adults. A placebo-controlled double-blind study.* J Clin Invest. 1996;97:1129-1134.

Zanarini MC. *Omega-3 fatty acid treatment of women with borderline personality disorder: a double-blind study.* Am J Psychiatry 2003;160:167-9.

Sangiovanni J. *Meta-analysis of dietary essential fatty acids and long-chain polyunsaturated fatty acids as they relate to visual resolution acuity in healthy preterm infants.* Pediatrics 2000;105:1292-8.

Salem N. *Mechanisms of action of docosahexaenoic acid in the nervous system.* Lipids 2001;36:945-59.

Zimmer L. *The dopamine mesocorticolimbic pathway is affected by deficiency in n-3 polyunsaturated fatty acids.* Am J Clin Nutr 2002;75:662-7.

Ikemoto A. *Reversibility of n-3 fatty acid deficiency-induced alterations of learning behaviour in the rat level of n-6 fatty acids as another critical factor.* J Lipid Res 2001;42:1655-63.

Seddon J. *Dietary fat and risk for advanced age-related macular degeneration.* Arch Ophtalmol 2001;119:1191-9.

Smith W. *Dietary fat and fish intake and age-related maculopathy.* Arch Ophtamol 2000;118:401-4.

Cho E. *Prospective study of dietary fat and the risk of age-related macular degeneration.* Am J Clin Nutr 2001;73:209-18.

Lauritzen L. *Fluctuations in human milk long-chain PUFA levels in relation to dietary fish intake.* Lipids 2002;37:237-44.

Makrides M. *Long-chain polyunsaturated fatty acid requirements during pregnancy and lactation.* Am J Clin Nutr 2000; 71:307-311.

Gibson R. *N-3 polyunsaturated fatty acid requirements of term infants.* Am J Clin Nutr 2000;71:251-5.

BIBLIOGRAPHY

Moriguchi T. *Recovery of brain docosahexaenoate leads to recovery of spatial task performance.* J Neurochem 2003;87:297-309.

Jensen G. *Effect of docosahexaenoic acid supplementation of lactating women on the fatty acid composition of breast milk lipids and maternal and infant plasma phospholipids.* Am J Clin Nutr 2000;71:292-9.

Cheruku R. *Higher maternal plasma docosahexaenoic acid during pregnancy is associated with more mature neonatal sleep-state patterning.* Am J Clin Nutr 2002;76:608-14.

Fan YY, Chapkin RS. *Importance of dietary gamma-linolenic acid in human health and nutrition.* J Nutr 1998; 128:1411.

Belch JJ, Hill A. *Evening primrose oil and borage oil in rheumatologic conditions.* Am J Clin Nutr 2000 Jan; 71(1 Suppl):352S.

Part 7: the omega-3 program

Kris-Etherton P. *Fish consumption, fish oil, omega-3 fatty acids and cardiovascular disease.* Circulation 106:2747-57.

De Lorgeril M, Salen P. *Diet as preventive medicine in cardiology.* Curr Opin Cardiol 2000;15:364-70.

Hu F. *Optimal diet for prevention of coronary heart disease.* JAMA 2002;288:2569-78.

Singh R. *Randomised controlled trial of cardioprotective diet in patients with recent acute myocardial infarction.* BMJ 1992;304:1015-9.

Singh R. *Effect of an Indo-Mediterranean diet on progression of coronary artery disease in high-risk patients.* Lancet 2002;360:1455-61.

De Lorgeril M, Salen P. *Dietary intervention in coronary care units and in secondary prevention.* In "Acute coronary syndromes. A companion to Braunwald's Heart Disease"/editor Pierre Théroux. Elsevier Science (USA) 2003; chapter 44:613-31.

Salonen J. *Intake of mercury from fish, lipid peroxidation, and the risk of myocardial infarction and coronary, cardiovascular, and any death in eastern Finnish men.* Circulation 1995;91 645-55.

Cahu C, Salen P, de Lorgeril M. *Farmed and wild fish in the prevention of cardiovascular diseases : assessing possible differences in lipid nutritional values.* Nutr Metab Cardiovasc Dis 2004;14:34-41.

Simopoulos A. *Common purslane: a source of omega-3 fatty acids and antioxidants.* J Am Coll Nutr 1992;11:374-82.

Simopoulos A. *N-3 fatty acids in eggs from range-fed Greek chickens.* N Engl J Med 1989;321:1412.

Renaud S. *Small is beautiful: alpha-linolenic and eicosapentaenoic acids in man.* Lancet 1983;1:1169.

Hu F. *Frequent nut consumption and risk of coronary heart disease in women: prospective cohort study.* BMJ 1998;317:1341-5.

De Lorgeril M. *Dietary arginine in prevention of cardiovascular diseases.* Cardiovasc Res 1998;37:560-563.

De Lorgeril M, Salen P, et al. *Potential use of nuts for the prevention and treatment of coronary heart disease: from natural to functional foods.* Nutr Metab Cardiovasc Dis 2002;11:362-71.

In our collection Alpen Éditions:

-The Omega-3 Answer

-Living with a Hyperactive Child

-All About the Prostate

-The French Paradox

-The XXL Syndrome

with Michel Montignac:

-Eat Yourself Slim

-The Montignac Diet Cookbook

-The French GI Diet

-Glycemic Index Diet

www.alpen.mc